Healthcare and Big Data

Mary F.E. Ebeling

Healthcare and Big Data

Digital Specters and Phantom Objects

palgrave
macmillan

Mary F.E. Ebeling
Drexel University
Philadelphia, Pennsylvania, USA

ISBN 978-1-137-50220-9 ISBN 978-1-137-50221-6 (eBook)
DOI 10.1057/978-1-137-50221-6

Library of Congress Control Number: 2016947279

Printed on acid-free paper

This Palgrave Macmillan imprint is published by Springer Nature
The registered company is Nature America Inc. New York

For the generations connected through me that have already gone
and that are yet to be.
But especially for Savannah (Mashashe) and Tim.

Acknowledgments

It was only through a series of what I call "alignments and coincidences" that this book came to be. In many ways, it demanded to exist. But this existential demand does not lessen the struggle that it took to bring it into material form or the deep appreciation that I feel toward all those who generously contributed to make this book a reality.

A series of alignments occurred in the spring of 2014 that made this all happen, including a residency that I participated in at the Department of Sociology at the University of Surrey (UK). Here, through the graciousness of people like Sara Arber and Nigel Gilbert, and especially Paul Hodkinson, who was my mentor, I developed the seed of this book in a scholarly environment rich in compassion, inspiration, and stimulating conversations. My gratitude extends to Geoff Cooper, Nicola Green, Susan Venn, Christine Hine, Mahamani Cronin, Agnes McGill, Ozge Dilaver Kalkan, and Rob Meadows. It was the bravery of others at Surrey who, in private conversations, shared their own stories of trauma around pregnancy loss and stillbirth that emboldened me to write this book. In their courage to express their pain, I found the strength to speak to other patients through the words that I write here. Laura Harvey, also at Surrey, set another alignment in motion when she led me to the organization Request Initiative, and to people like Margot Gibbs and especially Samir Dathi. I thank you for your generous help with a rather hopeless case. I must thank my dear and lovely friends Zoe Tenger and Tim Chitty for being my family in the UK, for keeping me warm and nourished on good conversations, nights knitting in front of the fire, for "pimping" my dinner, and for walks with Bubbles. Tim, I am especially grateful for the insights that you shared with me about the data industry and marketing, and for organizing meetings with data folks.

A coincidence that occurred within a few weeks of my return to the USA, an email from Lani Oshima, turned out to be significant to this book's existence. Without Lani's belief in the book, it would not have happened. Thank you Lani for your advocacy for this project.

Another alignment that made this book a reality happened through the generosity of Annemarie and Thierry Jutel. Thanks to you both for opening your home to me and teaching me about the Kiwi way of life. Annemarie, thanks especially for providing me with the intellectual space to develop this project. My thanks to all of the fantastic participants in the Critical Diagnosis Network at Victoria University of Wellington (New Zealand) who showed interest in this project and certainly my thanks extends to Kevin Dew (sociology, Victoria University of Wellington), who so kindly found a place in sociology for me during my time in New Zealand.

I must give my heartfelt appreciation to the nurses and doctors concerned with my medical care that I describe in parts of this book, especially Susan and Rhonda. Without your compassionate care and support throughout my time at the clinic, I think the experience of my miscarriages and subsequent hauntings would have been even more devastating than they were.

As a sociologist, I am continually amazed by the generosity of the various experts that I ask to help me understand an unfamiliar phenomenon or something that does not make sense to an outsider like me. Before I pick up the phone or send a request email, I imagine the person on the other end will think I am crazy to be interested in some seemingly obscure aspect about data, data privacy, medicine, or health and bio informatics. But I am so wrong, every time—most folks are not only willing but enthusiastic and excited to share with me their knowledge, their insights, and their perspectives; for this I am grateful. For their generosity and their patience, I thank Reed Gelzer and Dr. Deborah Peel of Patient Privacy Rights, Andrew Peterson, Debra Diener, Pam Law, Frank Pasquale, Tom Puglisi, Nicole Salemno, Anuj Shahani, Mike Sherwood, Adam Tanner, and Brian Weekes. My deepest gratitude goes to all of the anonymous health practitioners, data analysts, health informatics specialists, data brokers, and other professionals who agreed to be interviewed. Without your vital input I could not have written this book.

My love and gratitude goes as well to all my comrades in scholarship that know the suffering as well as solidarity that the process of writing can bring. Thanks to Franklin D. Cason, Caroline Chmielewski, Chiming Yang, Linda Kim, Rea Tajiri, Amy Slaton, Janet Golden, Erin Hurt, Amy Yuen, Timothy Lancaster Hunt-Cuticchia, Matt Hunt, Maura Cuffie, Blythe Boyd, Doug Popora, Michele White, Deb Carson, David Divita, Elaine Prewitt, and Louis Portlock for reading drafts of unformed thoughts, listening to my ramblings and incoherent ideas, and, above all, for believing that the germ would grow into something that could be shared with others, especially when I had my doubts. More so, you all believed that readers might even find themselves in my words. Much gratitude for this faith goes to Brent Luvaas.

To Rachel Ellis Neyra and Tsitsi Jaji, you all get a little extra thanks for your empathy, tenderness, and friendship, in addition to the poetic fierceness that you generously share with me. My thanks too goes to Julie Brownlie for our four-hour conversation in Glasgow; our discussions confirmed for me that I was on the right path.

I received much editorial support from Cathy Hannabach through her sharp eye and close reading of my jumbled text. Gregory Lang, research assistant extraordinaire, read countless patent filings, legislation, and other texts that can challenge even the toughest of researchers, to find new connections between laws and data industry practices. Thanks to Dina Abdel-Rahman, as well. All of this support given to my project would not have been possible without the help, in the form of financial support, from the College of Arts and Sciences at Drexel University. Many thanks as well for the visual conceptualization and design input from Jay Muhlin, Mauro Zamora, and Damon Locks. Rachel Krause and Elaine Fan, my editors at Palgrave Macmillan, deserve a special thank you for all of their support and guidance in shepherding this book through the entire publishing process, a process that many scholars find daunting. They have made it painless.

Finally, all of the good fortune and gratitude that I feel for Tim Portlock, my husband, can never be adequately expressed here. Through the telling of my own story of trauma and loss, Tim is allowing me to tell his as well. His trust in me to honor his own pain through the words that I write is something for which I will be forever grateful.

Contents

List of Figures

CHAPTER 1

Out of Death, a Birth

Phantom Data

The story of phantom data, of digital specters and data revenants, is a true story. It is a story born from and haunted by death, in which death is made lively through data's mobility. You could say that it is a hard-boiled ghost story. All of the noir elements are there: It opens with a grizzled detective who narrates the story in the first person, so that you are looking at the clues through her eyes. You (as her) are thrown into the middle of a conspiracy that you must get to the bottom of, no matter how dangerous the investigation may be. And since this is a noir, there is no doubt that it will get treacherous. There is also the ominous presence of a mysterious, shadowy figure that you catch glimpses of, maybe as they turn a corner, but you never get a good look at them, only hints that they are there. You are not quite sure exactly who they are, and whether they intend you harm or if they are trying to warn you of danger. There are clues, little crumbs of conveniently dropped information that lead you down warrens of dream-like menace and torment. As you dig deeper into the muck, the dead ends leave you ungrounded; you lose your center, and you become increasingly confused and uncertain, not only about who this mysterious person is, but also about who *you* are. By the end, through your stupidly naïve and agonizing pursuit to uncover the mystery and firmly grasp the truth, all you are left with is the brutal discovery that the conspiracy is much larger than you can comprehend, its complexity overwhelming and silencing.

M.F.E. Ebeling, *Healthcare and Big Data*,
DOI 10.1057/978-1-137-50221-6_1

The cruelest truth of all is that the mysterious person you were after was yourself, and worst of all, *you* were the intended dupe the whole time.

Where is the setting of this noir narrative—the rainy, dark streets of New York City? The sprawling, sun-bleached, desolate avenues of Los Angeles? No, this story unfolds in the data warehouses nestled in some of the remotest business parks and small towns across the USA. The characters of our narrative are distributed as bits of code in databases maintained by some of America's most secretive corporations, such as Little Rock, Arkansas-based Axciom and the internationally sprawling Experian[1] plc, which is headquartered in Dublin and has locations in thirty-eight countries.

So this is the story's setting. Now let us look at the death that starts out our narrative, because as we know, all good noirs start with a death.

A Curious Thing Comes a-Knockin'

What a curious thing is this?

As I stood in the foyer, my back to the opened door, the mail carrier Mr. Frederick rang the doorbell before I was even fully into the house. I still had my bag hanging from my shoulder and keys in my hand.

"Wow, Mr. Frederick, this is unexpected, but hey, I always like surprises."

I live in a mid-Atlantic city neighborhood where a lot of my neighbors have deep Southern roots and retain a form of politeness long forgotten in most other US cities. It is the type of place where I both know the last name of my mail carrier, and I greet him as "mister."

Mr. Frederick handed me the box with a friendly smile.

"Thanks, you have a good one," I said as I let the screen door slowly close.

"You too," replied Mr. Frederick. He turned and bounded down the front porch stairs to continue on his delivery route.

Looking down at the unexpected package in my hand, I closed the front door. I had just returned home from the first scan of my pregnancy. At six weeks, it was quite early, but given my age (I recently turned 42) and my history of miscarriages (two so far), Dr. Gaonkar, my doctor, was being cautious. I was enrolled in a clinical trial testing a new in vitro fertilization (IVF) drug that stimulates ovarian follicle growth, so Dr. Gaonkar also needed to collect data from the scan for the study's sponsor. As a patient, I was not told who it was, but I assumed the sponsor was a drug manufacturer.

I put down my bag and gave the box a closer look. It was a white cardboard package, wrapped around a smaller box. The return address read Similac, and the brand's marketing copy read: "Strong moms plan for great nutrition." I shook the box close to my ear. It sounded like liquid sloshing against the sides of thin aluminum cans.

Softly chuckling to myself, I thought how strange it was to receive a box of unsolicited baby formula samples on the very day that I saw the fetal stem of my baby, nestled in the darkness of the ultrasound screen at my doctor's office. How could the marketers possibly know that I was pregnant? A fleeting thought crossed my mind—"*Doctor Gaonkar*"—but I shook it out as quickly as it entered.

"A little early for this?" I murmured halfway under my breath, addressing the box.

What a wasted effort on Similac's part. I marveled at how incongruous and off-the-mark marketers are, over and over again. They just never get it right with me. I would never feed my baby formula, especially from the likes of Similac or, worse, Nestlé. Being the sort of professional detective that I am, I kept a vigilant eye on big conspiracies, especially ones that involve large syndicates taking advantage of the poor and disenfranchised, and baby formula-makers are well known for promoting formula to low-income mothers and mothers in developing countries, who can scarcely afford the expensive breast milk substitute or who have no access to safe drinking water to mix the powder with.[2] No, I thought to myself, when my baby is born, she or he will be nourished from my body, not from a can.

This baby was years in the making. Four years, in fact. Over that time, I had undergone twelve invasive medical procedures, including intrauterine insemination and several rounds of in vitro fertilization. After going into more than $25,000 in credit card debt to finance my many attempts to make a baby, I was now entangled in a clinical trial. This was my last option. During these attempts, every single clinical visit, procedure, lab result, and discussion with my doctor or her nurses was documented in an electronic health record kept for me in the clinic's computer, which is connected to the university medical system's larger database network. These data were transmitted to my health insurer, the pharmacy, and other businesses, such as the assisted reproduction financing company as well as the issuing bank of the credit card I used for co-pays and expenses not covered by insurance. When I told my doctor that my health insurance would not cover any of the IVF procedures, she offered me a brochure anced Reproductive Care, Inc. (ARC), a third-party business that elationship with fertility specialists and clinics, such as my doctor, to provide financing for IVF expenses (at a 14 percent interest rate). As a patient, I rarely thought of what happens to all of the data that was produced from my body, from my health status or even my ability to pay for my medical expenses that were all collected inside the doctor's office. I was too busy being a patient, and I assumed that the information was private and secure, and, therefore, protected. These digital pathways that my health data traversed have become the trails of investigation I now pursue as a detective.

Though I certainly did not feel lucky in regard to my infertility, from time to time, I did think about other patients who were facing much bigger challenges than I—I was not fighting to stay alive, I was only struggling to make a new life. The day the unsolicited baby formula samples arrived, though, I was feeling pretty lucky. After all this time and all the emotional turmoil and physical exhaustion that undergoing artificial reproductive medical procedures produces, there were two heartbeats in my body. Maybe I was under a baby spell that day, because if I had thought about it, I would have remembered that only a few months earlier, during a time when I was not pregnant after having suffered two miscarriages, I had received several taunting phone calls.

"Hello?"

"Congratulations on your pregnancy! I'm Marla from Allaboutthebaby.com and I want to talk to you today about some of our products and services that we can offer you as a …"

"I'm not pregnant." I cut off Marla's chirpy little spiel mid-sentence. The tears began to well up in my eyes.

"Uh, but the computer says you are."

Caught off guard, Marla was momentarily less chirpy. She sounded perturbed, not with the fact that she just caused a stranger anguish, but with the "they" that maintains the database that she is using to make the hundreds of autodialer phone calls during her shift that evening. "They need to update this."

"They do!" I screamed into the phone. I hung up.

Looking back now, how could I have known that in my sixth week of pregnancy there was a conspiracy in the works, with me ensnared in the center of its web? And later, standing on my doorstep, looking down at the odd delivery of an unsolicited box of baby formula, how could I have imagined that this piece of direct mail was, in fact, a ghoulish premonition?

Little did I know that I was about to be haunted by a tenacious phantom, for years to come. No, on that sunny February day I was too mesmerized, enthralled really, by the lively and lovely pixels that I had just witnessed on the ultrasound screen.

A week later in the doctor's office, the week seven scan produced a worried look on Dr. Gaonkar's face. As she stood in front of the monitor with her face in profile, I could see that she was counting the heartbeats under her breath. She said the heartbeat really should be about one hundred beats per minute, and she has counted only eighty. And the baby's growth seems to have stalled at six-and-a-half weeks. Nothing to worry about, really, she said. Though there are benchmarks, each baby develops on its own timescale. She faintly smiled and patted me on the shoulder. I held on to her offer of hope. Over the past four years, she had made many such offers.

Over the next week, I consciously ignored the signs. My breasts stopped hurting as much as they had been and the welcomed waves of nausea had subsided. More than the physical signals, I just "felt" that something, a presence I suppose, had left me. When my husband and I went to Dr. Gaonkar's office for another scan during the eighth week, the vibrating pixels were silent. The baby had died. My husband held my hand as I lay prone on the gurney, looked at me with wide eyes, and put his head on my breast. We cried together.

Through our crushing grief, my husband and I somehow left my doctor's office, hailed a taxi, and made our way home. Unlocking the door, he pushed against a pile of mail that Mr. Frederick had delivered earlier. Waiting for me on the top of the pile was the first issue of a complimentary year's subscription to *American Baby* magazine. I had not subscribed to the magazine. Through anger and tears, I summoned up my sleuthing skills, and tracked down the name and phone number of the subscription service that sent me the magazine. Dialing the 1–800 number I found on the masthead, I yelled at the hapless call center employee once I got through the maze of customer service button options.

"Can you let your bosses know, those marketing geniuses that they surely are, that my baby died today and I don't want their fucking magazine!"

"Uh oh. I am soooo sorry ... I will." I hung up before he could say another word.

On that horrendous day, I started to collect the clues for the hard-boiled noir that you now are reading. Over the months and years since I lost my baby in March 2011, I have received more than eighty separate email solicitations, social media advertisements, phone calls, mailed boxes of baby formula and diaper samples, magazines, baby photography offers, baby clothes, and direct-marketing flyers advertising everything from savings bonds to cord-blood banking. Much of the unsolicited mail I receive features softly lit photographs of dewy skinned babies, so freshly scrubbed I can almost smell the baby powder through the image, who beckon to me to buy Enfamil formula or a $1,200 Bugaboo All-Terrain stroller. The bulk of the direct mail offers, however, are for children's life insurance. I find these marketing offers particularly ghoulish.

One of the biggest clues, a real breakthrough for this detective, arrived in the mail on November 25, 2011, ten months after my final miscarriage. I received a letter from a local university research lab that focuses on early language development in infants. The letter invited me to bring my baby in to participate in some exciting new research focused on how infants acquire language before they start speaking. The letter closed with yet another invitation: "If you have any questions, call us!"

I called them. The lab manager, Eliza, answered the phone. I said: "I received your lab's letter and I would like to know, thank you very much, how you got my information. I am a sociologist who studies medicine and the pharmaceutical industry. I don't have a baby to bring in to participate in your study—I had a miscarriage ten months ago."

I was shaking a little.

Eliza gasped, which made my shaking subside a bit. "Let me look up the record right now."

Listening silently with my ear to the phone, I heard her tap the keyboard. She told me that they bought all of their recruitment databases from Experian, specifically a database called the *Newborn Network*. I thought to myself: "Wait, isn't Experian the company that runs credit reports? Why would they sell mailing lists and how do they have this erroneous information about me?" As this detective was to learn during her investigation, the *Newborn Network* was just the tip of the iceberg.

"So, we bought this database of new parents in a four-county area surrounding the university, and in the database, we have your name, mailing address, telephone number, and the birth month and year of your baby."

The shaking started again. "And what does it say, what is the birth date?"

"March 2011."

My marketing's baby birth date is the same as my fleshly baby's death. This letter became the most concrete clue that there is indeed a "mysterious person" out there, so essential to a noir narrative, and at the same time that there is a conspiracy underfoot. Now is this a coincidence? Any good detective worth her second-hand trench coat knows there are no coincidences.

My Marketing Baby, Born of Big Data

This book is about the conspiracies I uncovered through the pursuit of my baby—not my fleshly baby lost in the miscarriage, but my "marketing baby," born of big data in the distributed databases of marketers and data brokers. Much as the revenants in Stanislaw Lem's novel *Solaris* (1961), departed loved ones who are reanimated by the regrets of the living, that return to haunt the inhabitants of a space station orbiting a sentient planet, *data* revenants in the Age of Big Data come to haunt our everyday lives. Revenants are the dead that return to inhabit an uncanny life. They are not ghosts—they have bodies—but they are hollow bodies, puppet-like shells of the formerly living (Kilroy-Marac 2014, p. 256). Sometimes we ask them to come to us, such as when we fill in personal information on WebMD in exchange for health information. Other times, we consciously try to kill them, such as when we register our phone number on the national Do Not Call Registry. But either way, one cannot kill the undead, especially the digital undead. My data revenant takes the form of a marketing baby. For others, a data phantom may take the shape of a dead relative, such as was the case for Mike Seay, a grieving father who received a piece of junk mail addressed to "Mike Seay, Daughter Killed in Car Crash." For still others, a data phantom may take the figure of a health diagnosis embodied in advertising, like an HIV-positive man who receives online ads for antiretroviral drugs (Pearce 2014; Robertson and Pettypiece 2014).

In this book, I focus on how these data phantoms haunt health information in the USA. Such information is often assumed to be "private data," as it is produced by patients within digitized healthcare systems, but these data in fact go on to be innovated upon, packaged into new data assets, commodified and traded among data brokers. I focus on the process that private health information undergoes to become data commodities. I look at how innovation transforms health information from "dead" matter into "lively" data, and in the process, gives birth to both commodities and ownership claims. Throughout the book I consider how these interventions raise questions about what is considered public and private information, who may lay claim to data ownership and why, and how those tensions are exploited by US capitalist medicine and the health-care industries, especially those companies working in digital health.

My data revenant is a marketing baby that continues to live, while the other one died. My marketing baby lives an ersatz life made of algorithms, electrons, silicon crystals, binary code, and marketing images of what a middle-class "American Baby" is supposed to long for. A marketing baby is filled, overflowing, in fact, with desire. It is a thing that craves things: fat on processed foods, powdered milk, and overdoses of antibiotics; and clothed in disposable baby fashion that is stitched together by mothers paid pennies, who, in their desire for a better life for their own babies left with grandparents, work in precariously built factories in danger of collapse or fire, in places such as Dhaka or Ho Chi Minh City.[3] My marketing baby wants to go to Sears Portrait Studio, not strapped to a baby seat attached to my bicycle, but snuggled in an expensive car seat in a baby-safe SUV. My marketing baby demands that I save its umbilical cord blood to be cryogenically banked because in the future, medical science will be so advanced that doctors will be able to save its life by developing personalized medicine using its own stem cells. Over the years, my marketing baby has grown bigger, a baby who has surpassed toddlerhood and is now ready for pre-school. I know this because I receive online ads for school supplies and early learning software. It stomps its pudgy little feet and screams that I never buy enough for it. It keeps asking, very nicely and pretty please, to buy it things, and I never, ever listen. My marketing baby sticks out its lower lip in a pout and crosses its chubby arms. It screams to be listened to. It has an insatiable appetite for cheap consumer goods. My marketing baby lives a life of infinite consumption, of abundance, of endless consumer credit, of a desire for more and more and more. My marketing baby is an *enfant fatal*.

I decided awhile ago that if this baby was going to make such demands but refused to reveal itself to me, I mean really show itself, not just tease me with glimpses of itself through offers of Gerber Life Insurance policies ("The Grow-Up Plan") or free samples of Huggies diapers, that I would have to find it myself. I would go to the remotest data warehouses that it resides in and force this baby of algorithms, data mining, and mailing lists, demand that it come out of the shadows to face me—woman to thing—and explain itself. I would draw upon all my skills and perspectives that I have developed as a sociologist and apply them as a detective, bent on getting to the bottom of the "truth." Through my pursuit, I have found other women, and some men as well, also haunted by their own data revenants, marketing babies, and digital specters.

Soo-jin,[4] a woman in her mid-thirties living in a large US city with her toddler son and partner, noticed the ghostly visits in her third month of pregnancy. The hauntings were a trickle at first; her marketing baby barely whispered its desires. Coupons for diapers or an occasional cardboard flyer promoting studio portraits appeared in her mailbox. Later, Soo-jin received a deluge of offers, some more torturous than others. Ones that she found particularly disturbing were the brochures slipped into her mailbox for cord-blood banking. These bits of marketing communications, especially the ones concerning the future health of her unborn child, induced feelings of anxiety in her:

> I was wondering, wow they're really pushing this thing. I actually debated doing it [cord-blood banking] because I felt so much pressure because there was so much advertising about, you never know and to have that security. In the end, we didn't do it, but I just remember thinking that that was a little disturbing.

Soo-jin works as a senior administrator in a state university system, and, like most American workers, uses employer-sponsored health insurance as her primary medical coverage (Kaiser Family Foundation 2014). When she became pregnant with her son, she registered with a well-known university medical system close to her home. For each pre-natal visit, Soo-jin would place her hand in a biometric ID scanner at the registration desk and her electronic health record would come up on the nurse's computer screen. All of her data, her identifying information as well as her health data, were collected and entered into this electronic health record. For every visit, details about her health and the procedures performed by the doctor were coded, sent to the medical system's billing office, and then transmitted electronically to her health insurer for reimbursement. She assumed that hundreds of people must have seen some portion of her health record as her data travelled along the digitally networked route. She had a nagging suspicion in the back of her mind that some of her data had been leaked from the doctor's office to the marketers now contacting her. This worry was compounded by the fact that the cord-blood banking marketing brochure she had received at home was the same one that she saw in her doctor's waiting room.

Like mine, Soo-jin's age and other health factors meant that her pregnancy was considered high-risk. She had several genetic tests done in the first trimester. She suspects that some of the marketing materials that she received, especially the ones that seemed more "medically focused," also were connected to these tests. She also used her credit card to pay for all of the procedures related to her pregnancy, including the tests, health insurance co-pays for the pre-natal visits, and the prescriptions for medications. This is another possible connection. But she also suspects her data revenant was at least partially summoned by her own online and offline behaviors. After all, she had searched the web on several occasions looking for more information about what happens during pregnancy, and she had registered with retailers such as Destination Maternity, Diapers.com, and Babies 'R' Us. She had also used the customer loyalty card issued to her by Duane Reade, a retail pharmacy, whenever she purchased her prescriptions or over-the-counter items, such as pre-natal vitamins. In a certain way, she feels that she is ultimately "responsible" for the haunting by data marketers. Her data revenant took on a similar shape as mine, in the form of direct marketing concerning pregnancy and childbirth that appeared in her mailbox.

During my investigation, I came across an article in the *New York Times* Business section, about a woman, Marcy Campbell Krisk, who, like me, was haunted by a marketing baby, and has been so for ten years, after undergoing medical treatment for infertility (Freudenheim 2009). She told the journalist that the apparitions began soon after she had purchased fertility drugs at a retail pharmacy in her hometown. And as with my own marketing baby, Krisk's revenant aged through the direct marketing that she received, from newborn to toddler. She told the reporter that she suspected that the pharmacy had sold her health and identifying information to marketers. Krisk's story becomes another clue in my detective's tale.

I also found another woman, Ester, who experienced a haunting, but Ester's ghost hit much closer to home for this humble detective. Like me, she also started to receive visits from her data revenant while miscarrying her fleshly baby. She noticed that her baby started knocking at her door around the sixth week of pregnancy, after she had registered with Babycenter.com to use the site's due date calculator tool. She now believes that this is how her haunting started, which continued through four miscarriages:

> It's not surprising, like targeted advertisements as soon as you search for something on Google, it's pretty amazing. I can specifically remember sit-

> ting in the OB/GYN's office after my miscarriage one, two, and three, and thinking they should really have different waiting rooms for women who are undergoing a pregnancy loss, because it's just everything is so magnified at that time. These days I just throw away junk mail. Those days it was like I wanted to burn my mailbox.

After her fourth pregnancy loss, Ester went online and unsubscribed to all of the pregnancy websites that she had signed up for. Like Soo-jin, Ester felt that she, in some way, was responsible for the creation and summoning of her data revenant that took the uncanny form of targeted and personalized marketing.

With *Healthcare and Big Data,* my aim is to show how patients and users of healthcare in the USA are subject, with or without our consent, to massive data surveillance, collection, and commodification. Many Internet and information scholars have long linked Foucauldian concepts of panoptic surveillance and the biopolitics of categorization to massive data collection as a rationalization for social control (Beniger 1986; Elmer 2004; Lyon 1994). Yet, in the Age of Big Data and late capitalism, in which terabytes of digital information are produced, collected, and optimized on a daily basis, science and technology studies scholars have argued that our understanding needs to move beyond the panoptic governance of private health information. We need to understand how the process of commodification produces biovalue. In the case of healthcare, biovalue is the surplus value, the data produced from patient bodies and redistributed to health insurers, pharmaceutical makers, and direct marketers as *profit* they capture from bio-based data commodities (Rose 2007).

Yet, the data that these commodities are based upon are commonly considered to be "private" data. As I will show throughout this book, private data constitutes a legal fiction. Bioethicist and legal scholar Karla Holloway defines legal fictions as assumptions that are clearly false but made to live a truth through legislation. One obvious example of a legal fiction is adoption, in which biological kinship is severed and legal kinship is reconstituted through court documents (Holloway 2014). One less obvious example, and the one I explore in this book, is when regulatory regimes create laws mandating that private health data only be used in the service of our individual health, for public health purposes (such as reporting to the Centers for Disease Control and Prevention (CDC) in the case of communicable diseases), or for health research purposes that will benefit others who are ill. This constitutes a legal fiction, in which the law creates a special class of ostensibly protected data, but in social practice, these special protections are essentially meaningless (Allen 2011; Holloway 2014). Private health data has become a commodity that serves the interests of the medical and health industries, and ultimately, of capitalism, not of the patients that produce the data. Furthermore, it is important to understand that our relationships to our health data exist within a broader asymmetrical power relationship when it comes to the larger context of digital data. We know that we are on the short end of the stick every time we are asked to click "I Agree" to the terms of service when we want to download the latest version of iTunes or swipe our debit card at the grocery store. We know that "something" is happening to our data once we produce it, share it, or hand it over in exchange for access to healthcare, health information, or other services, but we don't know exactly "what" is happening to our data, how it is used, or who exchanges it (Brunton and Nissenbaum 2015). As information privacy and legal scholar Frank Pasquale describes it, the Age of Big Data constitutes a "black box society" in which most of us, even those of us who work within the data industry, as I demonstrate in Chapter 7, do not fully understand the algorithms and information networks that control, transmit, or analyze our data (Pasquale 2015).

In the wake of National Security Administration (NSA) whistleblower Edward Snowden's leaks proving that the US government collects massive amounts of data on US citizens and non-citizens alike, many of us have become jaded as regards any individual's ability to protect the privacy of her data, whether the data is produced online or not. By the time that Snowden was meeting secretly with journalists Glenn Greenwald and Ewen MacAskill and filmmaker Laura Poitras in a Hong Kong hotel room in early June 2013, the US Senate Committee on Commerce, Science, and Transportation (Commerce Committee) was compiling Congressional testimony and research on mass surveillance and data collection by the private sector, primarily by an obscure sector loosely characterized as "data brokers" (US Committee on Commerce, Science, and Transportation 2013; Gidda 2013; Poitras 2014). As I demonstrate in the following chapters, especially in Chap. 2, data brokers comprise a complex network of companies, ranging from well-established, publicly traded transnational corporations, such as Teradata Corporation and Experian plc, with their core business operations focused on information aggregation, data analytics, and data marketing services, to small, tech start-up subsidiaries that offer niche services, such as Slice, a software platform for online commerce that also collects and trades in consumer data (Slice Platform 2014). The collection and analysis of massive data by the private sector has one distinct difference from state data collection: The private sector's sole purpose in data collection is the innovation of new data commodities. While public sector bodies, such as the CDC or the Centers for Medicare and Medicaid Services, certainly do collect, trade, and share data, the law explicitly mandates that these data cannot be commodified. Data collected by government agencies cannot be innovated upon to be sold for profit—no money exchanges hands in any of the Data Use Agreements contracts that are made with the public sector.[5] Moreover, according to the very strict data use agreements between researchers who use datasets produced by public entities and the governmental bodies that hold them, ownership claims cannot be made by those who innovate upon the data. In fact, as Executive Order 13642: Making Open and Machine Readable the New Default for Government Information (2013) mandates, all data produced within the public sector must be made publicly available; it must be transparent (but secured by de-identification processes) and accessible, and the data are understood to be "owned" by the people (Burwell *et al.* 2013). The public sector considers itself merely the stewards of this data. For the private sector, however, data ownership is jealously guarded.

In response to Snowden's leak, there was broad outrage at governmental intrusions into our private lives, intrusions only made possible through the ubiquity of digital technologies. However, the more common and pervasive incursions by corporations and marketers garners much less attention.[6] Interestingly, this could be an indication not only that we know less about how private data brokers collect and sell our information, but also, despite having some awareness that it is happening, many of us are simply resigned to the fact that we are powerless to stop it, or at the very least, *believe* we are disempowered (Turow *et al.* 2015). My goal here is to explicate some of the reasons why so many of us feel hopeless in regard to controlling our health data by describing some of the ways our data is controlled and commodified by private industry.

This process of data collection, analytics, and commodification by the private sector constitutes a broader trend of big data, a term that has taken on a life of its own and is a shorthand way of describing both a process of data collection as well as a method to analyze large sets of information—anything from US Census data to quasar redshift rates in deep space, carbon emissions in a particular region, and to online click rates of users (boyd and Crawford 2012). Lately, big data is used to brand anything from business advice books (usually with the modifier "revolutionary"), to conferences, talk radio, healthcare summits, and television ads, even the title of this book that you read now. The term is everywhere, but its ubiquity says very little about what big data actually means for most of us. The phrase seems to be used predominately to sell the idea to the American public that somehow more data equals better results across most sectors of society, which in turn contributes to better lives for all of us. As a sociologist, I have written about how vested interests deploy this type of hyperbole when talking about new technologies, such as nanotechnologies (Ebeling 2008). The breathless predictions about how big data is going to change business and change our lives has a very familiar ring to it—most technological innovations tend to be touted as revolutionary by those who seek to make money from them. What exactly constitutes big data, and how it is impacting our lives, remains obscured. All we need to know, it would appear from the boosters, is that when big data is interrogated "smartly" by experts, it holds the answers to some of the biggest problems facing us in medicine, in business, and in life.

While large datasets historically have been collected on people, for instance in the form of census data or public health records, big data can be distinguished by what scholars and industry insiders call the four "Vs": Volume, variety, velocity, and veracity (Mehta 2015; Kobielus 2013). The amount of digital data globally has exploded exponentially in recent years, according to analyses by the International Data Corporation (IDC). In 2013, the digital "universe" consisted of more than 4.4 zettabytes (4.4 trillion gigabytes) of data, and it is expanding at a rate of about 40 percent a year (Turner *et al.* 2014). For our interests here, again in 2013, the volume of digitized *health* data globally reached 153 exabytes (153 billion gigabytes), and includes data from a variety of sources in the Internet of Things, such as networked medical equipment (EMC Corporation and International Data Corporation [IDC] 2014; Peterson 2015). This figure is set to grow at a faster rate than other forms of data as more health systems in Europe as well as in North and South America have been mandated to convert to digital record keeping (EMC Corporation and International Data Corporation [IDC] 2014). These data can include anything from magnetic resonance imaging (MRI) scans to YouTube videos and Twitter feeds, so volume necessarily indicates a variety, or diversity, of data as well—the second V that defines big data. The data can be scraped and collated from a variety of sources that are considered public, such as public records, as well as private, such as transactional data gleaned from a retailer.

Velocity of data, the third V constituting big data, means that data must be mobile for it to produce value. Data sitting on a server in a doctor's office only produces value once it is released to the payer, the health insurer or Medicare. Once in the data warehouses of a large insurer such as Blue Cross Blue Shield or Kaiser, then these data are reanimated and made to perform unimaginable feats through algorithmic physics. Only then can data be made to produce value, through its velocity. Finally, the fourth V, veracity, is in many ways connected to all the other Vs, since accurate and "clean" data (as it is called in the industry) is crucial to the reliability of big data; "bad" data will produce "bad" results.

I discuss at length how the large sets of health information that are collected, archived, and mined, and then mobilized, is only enabled by very powerful, distributed computing on a scale hardly imaginable until a few years ago. Digital media scholar Lev Manovich notes that big data derives its meaning necessarily from its tera- and petabyte sizes; data that are dually produced and analyzed by supercomputers and distributed computing power (Manovich 2012). He also notes that the meanings of big data shift as well with changes in computing technologies.

In particular, big data has taken on new meaning in the popular imagination since the *New York Times Magazine* published "How Companies Learn Your Secrets," an investigative article that uncovered how retailers, specifically *Target*, customize price markdowns to individual consumers by collecting data on in-store and online sales transactions and running predictive analytics on them, through this story big data came out of academic labs and into the popular imagination to take on new meanings of capitalist surveillance (Duhigg 2012). In fact, during my field work for this book, when I explained to participants that I was studying how information about our health is bought and sold by data brokers, only to come back to haunt us via direct marketing, many people replied, "Oh, just like the '*Target* Story.'" The *Target* story has become a way for many to contextualize and index the relationship between big data and healthcare. In contrast to the revolutionary promises made about the potentials of big data to improve our lives and health, big data often means mass surveillance and intrusions into what we consider to be private, and these data hauntings can have detrimental consequences for our health, our finances, and our lives (Mayer-Schönberger and Cukier 2012; Pasquale 2014). The confluence of big data and marketing surveillance produces some truly horrific stories: Facebook conducted "emotional contagion" psychological experiments on unsuspecting users without informed consent;

23andMe, a direct-to-consumer personal genetics company with financial links to both Google and Facebook, sold the "donated" health and genetic data of 800,000 customers to pharmaceutical companies for $60 million; and Apple's ResearchKit app collected health data on millions of iPhone users that was shared with researchers (Chen and Pettypiece 2015; Herper 2015; Regalado 2015; Kramer *et al.* 2014; Booth 2014). All these instances and many more demonstrate the skewed data bargains that people are forced to make every day. Through the following chapters, I examine the equally disconcerting trend of the private sector's wholesale collection of patients' health data from a variety of sources (marketers call this "cross-channel"), and the onward selling of patient health information to marketers.

The sleuthing legwork conducted in pursuit of my marketing baby has taken me to hospitals, government health facilities, and private clinics to interview health professionals who work with patient data on a daily basis. I spoke to these groups to understand how private health data moves from the doctor's office into the outside world. The investigation has taken me to database marketing conferences to speak with database marketers, data brokers, and data analysts. Collecting information from these subjects helped me understand how our personal health data is transformed into data commodities and used for all sorts of marketing and credit reporting within the health industry. I have participated in health privacy summits where I met with legal experts on privacy and patient data. I have interviewed financial professionals who handle data commodities, asking them how health data is collected from credit card and other financial transactions. I have spoken to pharmaceutical sales representatives who use prescribing data purchased from IMS Health Inc., the largest US-based health information data broker, to make sales calls to physicians. I have enlisted the help of other detectives, primarily those working in non-profit organizations concerned with data rights, information privacy and consumer protection, to help me in the pursuit of my "data subject"—the portfolio of information that has been collected about me and is held by data brokers. Finally, I have spoken to other patients who have been haunted by their own data revenants similarly constructed of dead material, bits of data, and, often, inaccurate information, that are released from databases into the world to clumsily stomp out a life of their own. But unlike the Creature in Mary Shelley's *Frankenstein,* these monsters are not seeking love and communion with humanity. Rather, they are searching for, demanding of, our money; they need us to buy for them consumer goods and things (Shelley 2003). Indeed, the actions of these data phantoms are much more akin to the execution apparatus depicted in Franz Kafka's *In the Penal Colony*, in which we, the condemned, have our crimes, or in this case, our data image, inscribed with rapidly vibrating and sharp needles on our skin, boring down over and over again, until the flesh falls from our bones (Kafka 2015).

In her book on the surveillance of Black lives, *Dark Matters: On the Surveillance of Blackness* (2015), Simone Browne analyzes the contemporary racialization of biometrics, apparent in current online sales of Black memorabilia, such as branding irons, used for enslavers' and slave traders' horrific practice of branding Black bodies with hot wires during the American slave trade, and indexes this to digital, racial profiling. Through this, she demonstrates how contemporarily what I call our "data images" brand our credit records, our health information, and our lives—they become part of who we are. Our data images replace our living, breathing selves. Whether or not these data images are accurate reflections of who we are or what we are facing in terms of our health, really does not matter in the eyes of marketers. The data revenants are released into the world with the knowledge that some of them will be successful and result in increased returns for marketers and their clients.

The Auto-ethnographic Noir

I opened this book with a first-person recounting of my initial confrontation with my data revenant in the shape of my marketing baby. In subsequent chapters, I start with similar narratives, set off at the beginning of each chapter to help distinguish them as an auto-ethnographic noir. As the primary ethnographic data that forms the basis of this research, I use my own experiences of healthcare, my own private health data that was breached, and my investigations into where and by whom my data is housed, commodified and sold, as well as my attempts to control my information and confront my marketing baby. Because these non-fictional stories are my recollections, it is important that these stories be distinguished from my sociological analysis. I did not, for example, have a voice recorder or a notebook in my doctor's office or when I received unsolicited marketing phone calls. These events are recounted as accurately as I can remember them, but they should not be considered "sociological data." Rather, they are illustrative of the social phenomena analyzed throughout the book. In these vignettes, I use the voice of a gumshoe, a narrative device exposing the links between academic social science research and noir detective work. Both types of investigations intend to master information, to get to the bottom of things. Yet, both often fail to produce definitive answers, instead inciting more ambiguity, more uncertainty and further investigations.

I take this approach to underline the situatedness of sociological knowledge, as well as my own positionality, to emphasize the black box of big data. Its allure and promise of total knowledge is a dangerous and false one, much like sociological research. We are all insiders and we are all subjects, including the data brokers that I interviewed, in the big data society. In the case of this book, that knowledge is situated in my body, in my data, and is under investigation. I often struggle with the notion of mastery. I am ambivalent toward the perceived need to master research methodologies, the "tools of my trade," or to master data or their analyses, as are many feminist social scientists that have influenced my approach (Haraway 1988). I am reluctant to develop a grand theory about "how it all works" and "what it all means," especially if it means placing myself somehow outside of the social phenomenon that I am theorizing. I am not alone in my ambiguity in this regard, as virtually every sociologist struggles with this. The detective of the noir genre, however, is a much more self-reflective and disenchanted observer. Just like a sociologist, the detective also relentlessly pursues mastery over information but from the opposite position of the researcher. The detective's life depends on it. It is her own story that is the mystery she is uncovering, whether she knows it or not, and by doing so, she may finally gain some control over the chaos. Yet throughout the pursuit, the gumshoe knows that she has an impossible task. Her attempts at mastery, at control, only lead to warrens of despair and obliteration—a hole that brings the detective to her own demise. The noir investigator always tells her story—in flashbacks—as the detective is dying or from the depths of her grave.[7] In the case of this book, these flashbacks are told not from the grave, but in the vignettes at the beginning of most of the chapters. Through using the auto-ethnographic noir approach, I underline the precarious relationship to knowledge to underline the futility and the impossibility of mastery.

In researching this book, this ambivalence about the sociologist's role has never been more poignant for me. It is an impossible task to expect of myself that I could understand the network that health data traverses in its entirety or in its complexity. I have found during my investigation that many of those who work in the industry do not understand it either, they do not understand the network's density nor can they chip through the opacity of the algorithms that produce and analyze the data, so how could I, as an outsider, do better than the professionals who work with health data day in and day out (Law 2004)? Again, the detective in a hard-boiled narrative accepts ambiguity, accepts the impossibility of total knowledge. In my pursuit as a sociologist, as a detective, and as an aggrieved mother of a marketing baby, I am drawn deeper into the morass. As I speak to more people, as I read more, as I investigate more, I become unmoored and adrift in the data ocean. What is the role of a sociologist anyway? Am I to explicate a system or to theorize it? Certainly with the succeeding chapters, I reveal nodes within the network: I analyze parts, such as specific companies, certain bits of legislation or concepts concerning data privacy; but to provide a thorough sociological explanation of its entirety is impossible. And that is the point. This is how the system that trades in our data, that silently intrudes into our private lives to profit, exerts hegemony. It needs to remain all encompassing, generally unnoticed, and utterly inexplicable to continue. This is how the NSA does it; this is how Experian does it.

This book is a document of my pursuit. In every chapter, I have included data that I collected from interviews and from work in the field. In all cases, I have promised those whom I have interviewed anonymity. All names that appear in the book are pseudonyms, and I do not name the cities where subjects live or work, nor do I use the names of their employers. The only identifying names that I use are those of brands, companies, and industry organizations. All participants who agreed to be interviewed were aware that I was a sociologist researching the use of private health data by data brokers.

I have been influenced by several other texts that employ auto-ethnography and narrative approaches to sociology, including *Ordinary Affects* by anthropologist Kathleen Stewart (2007), *The Vulnerable Observer* by anthropologist Ruth Behar (1997), *When Species Meet* by feminist theorist Donna Haraway (2008), *Motherhood Lost: A Feminist Account of Pregnancy Loss in America*, by anthropologist Linda Layne (2003) and *Testo Junkie: Sex, Drugs, and Biopolitics in the Pharmacopornographic Era* by philosopher Paul B. Preciado (2013). These books all have in common the utilization of a first person, affective narrative method of analysis that emboldened me to take on the auto-ethnographic noir approach with my own investigation. In Layne's ethnographic work on miscarriage, in particular, she places her body and the trauma of multiple pregnancy losses, especially in the opening chapter of her book, as the central pivot point for understanding maternal mourning practices and the affective networks that women build around miscarriage (Layne 2003, pp. 1–8). Sarah Polley's documentary film *Stories We Tell* has stayed with me for years since I first viewed it. Polley's deft recounting of her discovery that the father that she loves is not her biological father, told through interviews, speculative reconstructions, and flashbacks, is also influential in how I tell the stories laid out in this book (Polley 2012). In all of these books and in Polley's film, the researchers and filmmaker use their lives and bodies as their primary ethnographic sites and modes of analysis, expanding their analyses outwards from this embodied and affective position.

Chapter Descriptions

Documenting the detective legwork in my pursuit of my marketing baby, each chapter describes a key component or clue to uncover the mystery. In Chapter 2, I provide details concerning the data broker industry—those companies who trade personal consumer and health data. Chapter 3 describes data privacy, the US regulatory regimes that mandate the security of personal health information, and the networks that data traverses. Within this chapter, I explicate the core concepts of privacy, security, and consent. While in theory these concepts may ground data privacy legislation, in practice most privacy protection is a self-regulating mechanism run by the data industry itself; in essence, the wolves are guarding the hen house. Additionally, in the USA, privacy is legally regulated by sector and not by omnibus legislation (as data privacy is regulated in the European Union and a handful of other countries) (Singer 2013; Dyson *et al.* 2014). In the USA, data privacy legislation sprawls across many sectors of the economy, and includes statutes such as the Children's Online Privacy Protection Act (COPPA 1998), which protects the privacy of minors; the Health Insurance Portability and Accountability Act (HIPAA 1996), which regulates health data, the Fair Credit Reporting Act (FRCA 1970), that protects certain financial information; the Video Privacy Protection Act (VPPA 1988), which protects video rental customer data; and the Telephone Consumer Protection Act (TCPA 1991), which regulates telemarketing.

In Chapter 4, I show how data privacy and security is a social practice within clinical settings, through interviews with nurses, doctors, health practitioners, and public health researchers. In Chapter 5, I contrast these clinical rituals of privacy with the electronic health record industry, and the health data brokers that use software platforms and digital methods of capturing data and packaging it into innovative data assets, which undercuts the privacy work that health practitioners perform. In Chapter 6, the most theoretically exploratory of the book, I consider the shape of my marketing baby—what kind of life it embodies, especially as a data commodity fetish. Chapter 7 is a thick, ethnographic analysis of the empathy that this humble detective found at the Data Marketing Association's annual meeting. There I describe my hunt on the meeting's trade show floor and the unexpected result I found. Chapter 8 indicates what paths the investigation will take in the future, as all good noirs are indeterminate and open-ended in their final scenes.

And here, dear reader, I ask you to join me now in the following chapters on the quest for my marketing baby.

Notes

1. Since its 1996 merger with CCN, a UK company, Experian plc has been based in the European Union. Experian engaged in a reverse merger to take advantage of favorable corporate tax laws in Ireland. Reverse mergers have come under intense scrutiny during the Obama Administration, in large part because they allow US corporations to evade billions of dollars in US corporate taxes. As of January 2016, Experian plc had thirty-eight offices around the world.
2. Beginning in the 1970s, many women's health activists and international health organizations such as the World Health Organization have organized boycotts and other activism against Nestlé's aggressive marketing tactics, which include providing new mothers with samples of baby formula in hospitals, especially in developing countries (Moorhead 2007; Krasny 2012).
3. See the feminist literature on the historic feminization of labor within the global garment industry and the complex desires and reasons that motivate women to enter the industry (Siddiqi 2009).
4. All names of interviewees in this book are pseudonyms. I received ethics clearance for human subject research by Drexel University's Institutional Review Board (IRB), Protocol# 1409003104. The proper names of companies and brands are used, as they are registered with the United States Trademark and Patent Office, the Securities and Exchange Commission, or other entities.
5. While users of public data may be charged a fee for a download or for a data license, these fees are generally for the processing and packaging of datasets. They are not charged to make a profit off of the data.

6. The outrage seemed more intense at the time, since it revealed that the NSA continued its mass surveillance program with the approval and knowledge of the Obama Administration. While public knowledge of unwarranted wiretaps on US citizens was widespread during the Bush Administration, President Obama, as US senator and presidential candidate in 2008, had spoken out against the practice (notwithstanding the fact that he voted to renew the Foreign Intelligence Surveillance Act [FISA] in 2008) and had promised to strengthen privacy protections for US citizens once in office (Anderson 2008).
7. A common noir trope, especially within classic noir film, often opens with the investigator retelling the story of his death after the fact, in a first-person, past-tense voiceover that directly addresses the viewer. The aesthetic and narrative tropes I deploy in this book are considered in great detail by film scholars such as Naremore (1998) and Borde and Chaumeton (2002). Such narrative devices are evident in classic noir films such as *Double Indemnity* (1944), *Sunset Boulevard* (1950), and *Lady in the Lake* (1947).

References

Allen, Anita L. 2011. *Unpopular Privacy: What Must We Hide?* Oxford: Oxford University Press.

Anderson, Scott J. 2008. "Obama's Surveillance Vote Spurs Blogging Backlash." *CNN.com*, July 11. Accessed January 9, 2016. http://www.cnn.com/2008/POLITICS/07/11/obama.netroots/index.html?eref=onion.

Behar, Ruth. 1997. *The Vulnerable Observer*. New York: Beacon.

Beniger, James R. 1986. *The Control Revolution: Technological and Economic Origins of the Information Society*. Cambridge, MA: Harvard University Press.

Booth, Robert. 2014. "Facebook Reveals News Feed Experiment to Control Emotions." *Guardian*, June 29. Accessed January 9, 2016. http://www.theguardian.com/technology/2014/jun/29/facebook-users-emotions-news-feeds.

Borde, Raymond, and Etienne Chaumeton. 2002. *A Panorama of American Film Noir (1941-1953)*. San Francisco, CA: City Lights.

boyd, danah, and Kate Crawford. 2012. "Critical Questions for Big Data." *Information, Communication & Society* 15 (5): 662–79.

Browne, Simone. 2015. *Dark Matters: On the Surveillance of Blackness*. Durham, NC: Duke University Press.

Brunton, Finn, and Helen Nissenbaum. 2015. *Obfuscation: A User's Guide for Privacy and Protest*. Cambridge, MA: MIT Press.

Burwell, Sylvia M., Steven VanRoekel, Todd Park, and Dominic J. Mancini. 2013. "M-13-13 Memorandum for the Heads of Executive Departments and Agencies; Subject: Open Data Policy-Managing Information as an Asset." Memorandum, May 9.

Citizenfour. Dir. Laura Poitras. Praxis Films, Participant Media, HBO Documentary Films, 2014. Film.

Chen, Caroline and Shannon Pettypiece. 2015. "Apple's Health Research Kit Makes iPhone Users Test Subjects." *Bloomberg News*, March 9. Accessed July 1, 2016. http://www.bloomberg.com/news/articles/2015-03-09/apple-s-health-research-kit-makes-iphone-users-test-subjects.

Double Indemnity. Screenplay by Billy Wilder and Raymond Chandler. Dir. Billy Wilder. Paramount Pictures, 1944. Film.

Duhigg, Charles. 2012. "How Companies Learn Your Secrets." *New York Times*, February 19. Accessed January 9, 2016. http://www.nytimes.com/2012/02/19/magazine/shopping-habits.html?_r=0.

Dyson, Andrew, Jim Halpert, Thomas Jansen, Diego Ramos, Richard van Schaik, Scott Thiel, Carol A. F. Umhoefer, and Patrick Van Eecke. 2014. *Data Protection Laws of the World Handbook*. 3rd ed. Leeds, UK: DLA Piper.

Ebeling, Mary. 2008. "Mediating Uncertainty: Communicating the Financial Risks of Nanotechnologies." *Science Communication* 29 (3): 335–61.

Elmer, Greg. 2004. *Profiling Machines: Mapping the Personal Information Economy*. Cambridge, MA: MIT Press.

EMC Corporation, and International Data Corporation (IDC). 2014. "The Digital Universe: Driving Data Growth in Healthcare." Vertical Industry Brief: Healthcare. EMC Digital Universe. Hopkinton, MA: EMC Corporation. https://www.emc.com/analyst-report/digital-universe-healthcare-vertical-report-ar.pdf.

Freudenheim, Milt. 2009. "And You Thought a Prescription Was Private." *The New York Times*, August 9, sec. Business, BU1.

Gidda, Mirren. 2013. "Edward Snowden and the NSA Files: Timeline." *Guardian*, August 21. Accessed January 9, 2016. http://www.theguardian.com/world/2013/jun/23/edward-snowden-nsa-files-timeline.

Haraway, Donna. 1988. "Situated Knowledges: The Science Question in Feminism and the Privilege of Partial Perspective." *Feminist Studies* 14 (3): 575–99.

———. 2008. *When Species Meet*. Minneapolis: University of Minnesota Press.

Herper, Matthew. 2015. "Surprise! With $60 Million Genentech Deal, 23andMe Has a Business Plan." *Forbes*, January 6. Accessed January 9, 2016. http://onforb.es/1wRSbZX.

Holloway, Karla F.C. 2014. *Legal Fictions: Constituting Race, Composing Literature*. Durham, NC: Duke University Press.

Kafka, Franz. 2015. *In the Penal Colony*. Seattle, WA: Amazon Digital Services.

Kaiser Family Foundation. 2014. "Recent Trends in Employer-Sponsored Insurance." *JAMA* 312 (18): 1849.

Kilroy-Marac, Katie. 2014. "Speaking with Revenants: Haunting and the Ethnographic Enterprise." *Ethnography* 15 (2): 255–76.

Kobielus, James. 2013. "Measuring the Business Value of Big Data." *IBM Big Data and Analytics Hub*, May 9. Accessed January 9, 2016. http://www.ibmbigdatahub.com/blog/measuring-business-value-big-data.

Kramer, Adam D. I., Jamie E. Guillory, and Jeffrey T. Hancock. 2014. "Experimental Evidence of Massive-Scale Emotional Contagion through Social Networks." *Proceedings of the National Academy of Sciences* 111 (24): 8788–90.

Krasny, Jill. 2012. "Every Parent Should Know the Scandalous History of Infant Formula." *Business Insider*, June 25. Accessed January 9, 2016. http://www.businessinsider.com/nestles-infant-formula-scandal-2012-6#ixzz3kzLCYQa9.

Lady in the Lake. Dir. Robert Montgomery. Metro-Goldwyn-Mayer Studios, 1947. Film.

Law, John. 2004. *After Method: Mess in Social Science Research*. London: Routledge.

Layne, Linda L. 2003. *Motherhood Lost: A Feminist Account of Pregnancy Loss in America*. New York and London: Routledge.

Lem, Stanislaw. 1961. *Solaris*. Krakow: Pro Auctore Wojciech Zemek.

Lyon, David. 1994. *Electronic Eye : The Rise of Surveillance Society*. Minneapolis: University of Minnesota Press. http://site.ebrary.com/lib/drexel/docDetail.action?docID=10159374.

Manovich, Lev. 2012. "Trending: The Promises and the Challenges of Big Social Data." In *Debates in the Digital Humanities*, edited by Matthew K. Gold and Lauren F. Klein, 504. Minneapolis: University of Minnesota Press. http://manovich.net/index.php/projects/trending-the-promises-and-the-challenges-of-big-social-data.

Mayer-Schönberger, Viktor, and Kenneth Cukier. 2012. *Big Data: A Revolution That Transforms How We Work, Live, and Think*. Boston, MA: Houghton Mifflin Harcourt.

Mehta, Pankaj. 2015. "Big Data's Radical Potential." *Jacobin*, March 12. Accessed January 9, 2016. https://www.jacobinmag.com/2015/03/big-data-drones-privacy-workers.

Moorhead, Joanna. 2007. "Milking It." *Guardian*, May 17. Accessed January 9, 2016. http://www.theguardian.com/business/2007/may/15/medicineandhealth.lifeandhealth.

Naremore, James. 1998. *More Than Night: Film Noir in Its Contexts*. Berkeley: University of California Press. http://www.library.drexel.edu/cgi-bin/r.cgi?url=http://search.ebscohost.com/login.aspx?direct=true&db=nlebk&AN=42280&site=ehost-live.

Pasquale, Frank. 2014. "Reedescribing Health Privacy: The Importance of Information Policy." *Houston Journal of Health Law & Policy* 14: 95–128.

______. 2015. *The Black Box Society: The Secret Algorithms That Control Money andInformation*. Cambridge, MA: Harvard University Press.

Pearce, Matt. 2014. "Dad Gets OfficeMax Mail Addressed 'Daughter Killed in Car Crash.'" *Los Angeles Times*, January 19. Accessed January 9, 2016. http://articles.latimes.com/2014/jan/19/nation/la-na-nn-officemax-mail-20140119.

Peterson, Andrea. 2015. "Connected Medical Devices: The Internet of Things-That-Could-Kill-You." *Washington Post*, August 3. Accessed January 9, 2016.

https://www.washingtonpost.com/news/the-switch/wp/2015/08/03/connected-medical-devices-the-internet-of-things-that-could-kill-you/.
Preciado, Paul B. 2013. *Testo Junkie: Sex, Drugs, and Biopolitics in the Pharmacopornographic Era*. Kindle. New York: Feminist Press.
Regalado, Antonio. 2015. "Apple Has Plans for Your DNA." *MIT Technology Review*, May 5. Accessed January 9, 2016. http://www.technologyreview.com/news/537081/apple-has-plans-for-your-dna/.
Robertson, Jordan, and Shannon Pettypiece. 2014. "They Know You Buy Viagra and They Want to Sell You More." *Bloomberg Business*, December 10. Accessed January 9, 2016. http://www.bloomberg.com/news/articles/2014-12-10/they-know-you-buy-viagra-and-they-want-to-sell-you-more.
Rose, Nikolas. 2007. *The Politics of Life Itself: Biomedicine, Power, and Subjectivity in the Twenty-First Century*. Princeton, NJ: Princeton University Press.
Shelley, Mary. 2003. *Frankenstein: Or the Modern Prometheus*. London: Penguin Classics.
Siddiqi, Dina M. 2009. "Do Bangladeshi Factory Workers Need Saving? Sisterhood in the Post-Sweatshop Era." *Feminist Review* 91: 154–74.
Singer, Natasha. 2013. "Data Protection Laws, an Ocean Apart." *New York Times*, February 3. Accessed January 9, 2016. http://www.nytimes.com/2013/02/03/technology/consumer-data-protection-laws-an-ocean-apart.html.
Slice Platform. 2014. "Slice Platform Lets Partners Create Engaging and Personalized Shopping Experiences." Press Release. Palo Alto, CA. http://www.reuters.com/article/2014/09/11/idUSnMKWWxZ2xa+1e8+MKW20140911#y7a2itjpfJ4Wo6oM.99.
Stewart, Kathleen. 2007. *Ordinary Affects*. Durham, NC: Duke University Press.
Stories We Tell. Dir. Sarah Polley. National Film Board of Canada, 2012. Film.
Sunset Boulevard. Screenplay by Charles Brackett and Billy Wilder. Dir. Billy Wilder. Paramount Pictures, 1950. Film.
Turner, Vernon, John F. Gantz, David Reinsel, and Stephen Minton. 2014. "The Digital Universe of Opportunities: Rich Data and the Increasing Value of the Internet of Things." White Paper 1678. EMC Digital Universe. Hopkinton, MA: EMC Corporation and International Data Corporation (IDC). http://idcdocserv.com/1678.
Turow, Joseph, Michael Hennessy, and Nora Draper. 2015. *The Trade-off Fallacy: How Marketers Are Misrepresenting American Consumers And Opening Them Up to Exploitation*. A Report from the Annenberg School for Communication University of Pennsylvania. Philadelphia: University of Pennsylvania.
US Committee on Commerce, Science, and Transportation. 2013. *A Review of the Data Broker Industry: Collection, Use, and Sale of Consumer Data for Marketing Purposes*. Washington, DC: Office of Oversight and Investigations. http://www.commerce.senate.gov/public/?a=Files.Serve&File_id=0d2b3642-6221-4888-a631-08f2f255b577.

CHAPTER 2

The Rise of the Databased Society

"If you would like to participate, or would like more information, please call us." The letter from the infant language lab turned out to be one of the biggest clues in helping me track down my data revenant, my marketing baby. The unsolicited correspondence is also the piece of hard evidence that indicates there is, indeed, a conspiracy underfoot. More than three years after my initial conversation with Eliza, the lab manager, I decided to call back. I still had questions about where my baby lived: Was it still residing in Experian's data warehouse or had it moved? How much did the lab pay Experian for my data? What was the price tag of my trauma and pain, exactly? Perhaps Eliza could help me understand.

With that letter inviting me to have my "baby" participate in a study, this humble detective was given a break.

"Hello, Eliza, I'm not sure if you remember me, but I called you a few years ago about how your lab got hold of my information, on a baby that I miscarried."

"Oh, yes, I remember you," Eliza said without hesitation, adding "And in fact, after we talked, I told Dr. Swanson, the head of the lab, all about what happened to you. We were hoping you'd call back."

Eliza's concern about my pain was reassuring; despite never having met her, throughout the faceless phone call, I pictured Eliza's features softened by the empathy I hear in her voice. I thought to myself "I have found the first ally in my quest." She answered my questions as I heard her click on the files in her hard drive.

M.F.E. Ebeling, *Healthcare and Big Data*,
DOI 10.1057/978-1-137-50221-6_2

Yes, they purchased a database of "new parents" living in a five-county radius of the university. It contained about 3000 names and the lab paid about $800 for it. But, Eliza warned me, you should know something.

"Well, while I told you that the database is 'owned' by Experian, we actually purchased the database through a New Jersey-based operation called the American List Counsel, the ALC."

"Uh, hum," I slowly responded, trying to process this new development. "Another company, A-L-C?"

"Yes. Do you want the names of the ALC sales force that I've dealt with?" Eliza read out the names, email addresses, and direct phone numbers of the ALC representatives that she regularly worked with to purchase databases. I wrote them down in my tattered detective's notebook.

As Eliza told me, she thought that most of the names that the ALC compiles comes from things like catalogs or memberships, she assumed that the people who are contained within the *Newborn Network* had knowingly registered, in some way, to receive more information and marketing for things related to babies.

For their purposes, the lab tries to purchase databases that only include residents identified to have a newborn child living in the household within the three surrounding counties. Some lists can include upwards of thousands of contacts, but generally most databases contain between 1 and 200 names and addresses, which are sorted by the month and year of the child's birth. For recruitment purposes, the lab tends to target parents of babies that are newborn to eighteen-months old. While she explained this, Eliza looked up the last invoice that the lab received from ALC, for a database purchased in November 2014: $800.00 for about 3000 area contacts.

"You know, none of us want something like this to happen. We're never sure if this is the best way to recruit participants, anyway," Eliza said before we hung up, and added, "Can you let us know what you find out?"

I promised her that I would report back anything I learn to them.

The conspiracy had just deepened. The ALC is what is known in the data industry as a "list broker" and the company's signature product is the "Newborn Network," a list that they put together with data that is "owned" by Experian Marketing Services, an arm of Experian plc (Magill-Cook 2015a, b).

How is it that the lab came to be in possession of such detailed, if inaccurate, information about my traumatic health experiences, and through a purchased database from two companies that I had never had direct contact with? How did my "baby" come to reside in the database warehouses of Experian or in, of all places, Princeton, New Jersey, the headquarters of ALC? I suspect that I am not the only one to have this impression, but I had thought of Experian as a consumer credit-reporting agency, one of the largest in the USA, which provides your bank with a history of your credit behavior when you apply for a loan or a credit card. As this detective learned through her investigations, however, Experian is so much more than just a credit bureau; it is one of the most powerful information brokers in the world that, through its ownership claims over consumer information, can determine whether someone can have a home, or a job, or even who may receive healthcare. I had never even heard of ALC nor of the term "list broker" (indeed, "data broker" was an unfamiliar phrase as well), but I could guess what these companies did for a living. How could a small research institute at a private university be allowed to purchase data on me, sensitive data that I had (falsely) considered my private health information, to market to me? How could a little known industry have so much power over my personal information? I had to investigate. I made a plan to call ALC to get to the bottom of this. Little did I realize at the time, far from finding an answer, much less my marketing baby, I was about to go down one of the many "Big Data warrens" that I found during my investigation.

An Industry You've Never Heard Of

Data brokers, sometimes referred to as data aggregators, information resellers, or database marketers, are companies in a variety of sectors that collect, collate, analyze, and profile individuals' personal information. Through this process, data brokers create new data commodities that are traded and sold, usually business-to-business. The data broker industry is multilayered and complex; most brokers buy and sell data among themselves, and many companies do not identify as "data brokers" whatsoever, since the collecting and selling of data is not their core business. For those corporations whose core business is the trade of data, most do not have contact or direct business relationships with consumers. Much of the data collection goes on without the knowledge or the expressed consent of most consumers (Federal Trade Commission 2014, p. 46).[1] Data brokers take public and private information, aggregate it into products, and monetize it. In short, brokers transform data into immaterial commodities that are bought and sold. Brokers package these data commodities through various innovations, which are almost always algorithmic interventions. Some of these algorithms are patented or proprietary. For instance, Experian Marketing Services owns more than thirty software and database patents, and others are licensed, or can be open sourced.[2] Data brokers then distribute these new commodities through data use or licensing agreements, or through the outright sale of data products to third-party companies like Nestlé, owner of *Gerber* baby and toddler nutrition products, or Mead Johnson, the makers of Enfamil, two of the many companies to directly market to me. This is what happened with the products created from my data. These clients then use these data products for any number of purposes that may include direct marketing, conducting background checks, helping make trade decisions on financial markets (this is often called by data marketers as "decisioning" on "actionable" data), innovating new consumer products, or preventing fraud. Data brokers obtain consumer information from diverse sources, including public records such as birth records, driver's licenses, and construction permits, as well as non-public information such as offline purchases you have made using a credit card, warranty cards that you may have filled out when making a purchase, and the billions of browser cookies your searching and purchasing behavior online has produced. Once these data are collected, secured, and transformed into new, segmented products, they become the data assets of data brokers. Through the combination of data possession and innovations, data brokers claim ownership of our data.

Companies that collect, aggregate, and sell consumer information to retailers, manufacturers, service providers of various stripes, financial institutions, healthcare providers, non-profit organizations, including educational institutions, law enforcement, and other governmental agencies may all be considered data brokers in that they collect data on their clients or customers and potentially can trade that data. Data brokers may also be credit bureaus, such as Experian or TransUnion, or advertising and marketing firms, especially database marketers like Digitas Health LifeBrands, a member of the global marketing and advertising firm Publicis Groupe. Virtually every social media platform or web-based information technology company—the Facebooks and the Googles of the world—are data brokers. Many of these companies invented the freeware model, or at least perfected it and turned it into a billion-dollar enterprise—where in exchange for the use of "free" online platforms, users and their data become the commodity that is sold to advertisers and marketers. Retailers themselves, from big box chains such as Target or Walmart, to smaller retailers may also be data brokers. When a grocery store gives the pers a "loyalty card," and then sells the data on customer pu. behaviors to another business, say an automobile insurer that uses this purchasing data for "price optimization" (a fancy way of describing the algorithms that collate seemingly unrelated data on an individual), that grocery store becomes a data broker (Samilton 2015).

In his book *What Stays in Vegas* (2014) Adam Tanner, a journalist who researches the use of personal data by the private sector, demonstrates the ways that casinos, as well, have become data brokers. Their data strategies include the use of loyalty or points programs that offer small discounts throughout a casino (casino restaurants, for example, will list two prices for menu items: discounted prices for loyalty cardholders, regular prices for non-cardholders) in exchange for access to a patron's gambling and consuming behavior throughout his or her visit. Large casino groups, such as Caesars Entertainment Corporation, also offer branded credit cards, following companies in other sectors, such as air travel, that use credit cards as both new revenue streams and new data streams. The Caesars Total Rewards VISA credit card, for instance, enables the casino to track cardholders' purchases not only at rival casinos but also at the grocery store, the gas pump, and, of course, online. Caesars uses these data to augur the individual consumer, in order to more precisely market to them, and to ensure that they keep coming back to Caesars.[3]

Public sector organizations may also act as data brokers. For example, in most states, the Department of Motor Vehicles (DMV) routinely and legally sells data, including driver's names, addresses, vehicle registrations, and the models of cars registered. The DMV can and does sell virtually all of the data that it collects on individual drivers (Sheer and Beladi 2015, pp. 58–59). Many public and governmental bodies, such as the Centers for Disease Control and Prevention, the National Institutes of Health, the Veterans Health Administration, the Centers for Medicare and Medicaid Services, and others, trade in large datasets that are produced and collated from disparate sources either within these public entities, or from other data sources, including electronic health records (EHR) software companies. A public health researcher, Sharon Wise, explained during my interview with her that many of the datasets that she uses in her research come from EHR companies that sell anonymized health records collected through digital healthcare platforms used in both public and private institutions, mainly hospitals. Larger EHR companies, such as Epic Systems Corporation, provide clients with health data analytics services performed on the in-house data collected through the Epic platform. On the whole, however, public entities are not in the business of commodifying data, as these data are considered "owned" by citizens and tax payers. Rather, these forms of public information are traded and shared through data use agreements, which, especially in the case of health information (discussed in the following chapters), have very strict protocols for how the data should be secured, stored, used, and disseminated by the third-party researcher that obtains these data. Depending on the type of data (financial, health, etc.), these agreements fall under the regulatory regimes of legislation such as the Gramm-Leach-Bliley Act (GLBA) or the Health Insurance Portability and Accountability Act (HIPAA).

The sale of data assets is not limited to business-to-business transactions; government entities also purchase large datasets from data brokers. The Transportation Security Administration (TSA), for instance, created their PreCheck prescreening program in 2011. The program offers travelers the option to pay $85 to voluntarily submit to a background check every five years in order to skip a lot of the security procedures at airports. The background check is performed by the TSA through the data surveillance resources made available by the Department of Homeland Security. Some of those resources include data and analytics from commercial brokers (Sheer and Beladi 2015, p. 59). Just before the Congressional holiday break in December 2014, the TSA quietly requested proposals from data brokers to expand the reach of their PreCheck surveillance to include social media, commercial information, and other publicly available data. Through the proposed expansion, the TSA promised to hand over all program analytics to the commercial sector (Corrin 2015). When news outlets reported on the TSA's plans, public outrage was swift, and the agency eventually withdrew the request for proposals within two months of its announcement. It became possible, because it was a case of government surveillance that the public—still reactive to the Snowden leaks about the National Security Administration (NSA)—was quick to respond and demand a shutdown of the request for proposal (RFP). These types of trades in private data happen every day by the corporate sector and go on without much of a public response.

Despite these examples of data trading by public entities, the bulk of the data broker industry comprises those companies whose core business is the collection, analytics, and sale of big data (Federal Trade Commission 2014; Barocas and Nissenbaum 2014). Many data brokers specialize in not only the collection, aggregation, and sale of data, but also offer innovative data management platforms—scalable software. Built out of highly sophisticated analytics, such platforms allow clients to scrape, store, analyze, and use data in meaningful ways for their businesses. For our interests here, for instance, Experian plc offers hospitals and other healthcare providers a risk assessment and data management platform, Experian Health, that allows a hospital to perform credit checks (among other functions) on admitted patients.[4] ALC, the list broker that your detective discovered was an attendant at the birth of my marketing baby, offers a data product to marketers, the Mh2 PrecisionBase Ailment Masterfile, a prospects list that combines the credit scores of consumers with their health information, including data from insurers such as Blue Cross Blue Shield (Steel 2013a; American List Counsel Inc. 2015). In sum, data brokers are in the big business of big data.

Where Do the Data Come From?

Data brokers collect personal identifiable information on consumers from more than 50,000 sources, which results in close to 70 billion bits of data held every year in database warehouses. These data are then aggregated, packaged into records that equates in about 200 records for every citizen in the USA, by far the largest number compared to other countries (Urbanski 2015). Emily Steel, a journalist specializing in consumer data for the *Financial Times* calculated that in 2013 an individual's personal information, such as their gender, mailing address and age, was worth less than $1, most personal consumer profiles garner less than a few cents, with more intimate information, such as health diagnoses or prescriptions that an individual may have fetching much more, but still under a $1 per record (Steel 2013b). Yet, when these records are in aggregate, they can be worth millions to the industry.

Data brokers collect information on us from three broad categories: public records, publicly available information, and non-public sources. What constitutes a public record is defined by local, state, and federal laws, and through the Freedom of Information Act (FOIA); most public records are generally accessible either online or made available on paper by request. Public records can include information that is produced through court proceedings such as criminal and prosecution records, court judgments, civil cases, lawsuits, property deeds, tax liens, and bankruptcy filings. Public records can also include construction permits; records of births, deaths, marriages, and divorces; voter registration forms (which may include party affiliation); and driver's licenses and other forms of state identification—virtually any data that is recorded with a local or state official. Publicly available information is data that while not a public record per se, is still freely accessible and not confidential, such as telephone directories, classified advertisements, and information from newspapers, magazines, websites, and other public sources. The founder of Infogroup, one of the most powerful data list brokers in the industry, Vinod Gupta, got his start by compiling Yellow Pages listings into customized lists for sale to marketers (Angwin 2015; Tanner 2014).

Non-public information derives from proprietary sources and its trade is usually contracted through data usage and licensing agreements made between a business or a data source and a data broker. Non-public data can include financial transactional data (including transactions made by consumers using credit and debit cards); information derived from customer loyalty cards used at retailers, pharmacies, or grocery stores; gift cards; warranty registrations; surveys; website registrations; deleted or incomplete posts on social media that are collected by the platform; browser histories and cookies; mobile phone tracking and usage; metadata; online purchases; and online searches.

When I contacted the ALC to learn more about their Newborn Network list product and how Experian was connected to the list, the executive vice-president who was in charge of the product explained that Experian used more than 50 sources to aggregate data on expectant parents, and considered these sources proprietary (Magill-Cook 2015b). She did not even know what the data sources were, the main ingredients that fed the *Newborn Network*, the ALC's most successful data product. Once the data owned by Experian was integrated into the *Newborn Network* databases, she told me that the information would "age" with the pregnancy and the newborn, for 18 years. Once these data are collected, secured, and transformed into new, segmented products, they become the data assets of data brokers, much like the ALC's lists and direct marketing products.

It is through these data assets that brokers own, that they are able to build complex and very detailed, albeit flat, marketing images of us all. These "data images" are constructed algorithmically across databases. Acxiom Corporation, based in Little Rock, Arkansas, for instance, is currently one of the largest data brokers in the USA and has a powerful global presence. The company describes itself as an "enterprise data, analytics and software-as-a-service company" (Acxiom Corporation 2015a). During 2015 alone, the company's database warehouses processed an average of

1 trillion data transactions per week on more than 700 million global consumers (US Committee on Commerce, Science, and Transportation 2013, p. 12; Acxiom Corporation 2015b, p. 9). This means that the company's data warehouses contain nearly 1500 data points on each individual they track (Singer 2012). These consumer profiles are often repackaged into direct marketing databases, with the high probability of an individual consumer being placed into fine-grained, targeted customer segment. These segmentations are then sold to any client that has the money to purchase the records. As I have already shown, these data are routinely sold usually to virtually anyone who can afford the purchase price, including the infant language research lab that contacted me.

Some data can derive from "internal" sources or clients of data brokers, in which case the information is harvested to produce new sources of value for the brokers. One of the most data-rich sources derives from credit worthiness platforms, such as Experian's credit reporting software platform. In my interview with credit union loan officer Paula Larson, she described how by law, all financial institutions must conduct a credit background check on potential customers who are seeking a loan, mortgage, or line of credit. Since there are only a few credit bureaus, with Experian, TransUnion, and Equifax being the largest, the credit bureaus have the economies of scale to provide sophisticated data platforms to clients. These platforms enable financial institutions to not only conduct financial risk assessments on customers but also input new data that is collected by the credit bureau free of charge. As Larson explained, the Experian credit risk services license agreement required her credit union to hand over new information on the applying clients in exchange for the credit union's use of the Experian platform—in other words, Experian gained more data without having to gather or pay for it directly. In fact through the use of Experian's credit reporting software platform, it is able to collect billions of data points on millions of individuals globally, as it operates in 38 countries (as of 2016), and these data become the raw material for the marketing services arm of Experian. Through Experian Marketing Services, the information company offers a marketing platform to clients that are seeking to target their customers, or potentially acquire new ones, by targeting them directly with more accurate and relevant marketing messages. One of the products that Experian offers are databases of consumers that have a "life-event trigger," which they define as the purchase of a new home, or the birth of a baby or a move to a new location. Clients can purchase highly customizable databases to fit their marketing needs. It was Experian's *Life-Event Trigger—New Parents* database that your detective believes directly fed into the ALC's *Newborn Network* database (Experian Marketing Services 2016).

Data collected by clients through direct marketing platforms becomes another source that brokers use to collect and aggregate data and to create new data products to be sold to clients, oftentimes the very clients that the data was sourced from to begin with. As one analyst who works for a broker explained it to me, these products are sold back to clients for "decisioning," or to help clients make choices about when to buy or sell securities, for example, or whether or not to give a bank customer a line of credit.

It is this process of data aggregation and analytics that data brokers, such as Acxiom or Experian, claim is the innovation, the "value-add" that they provide to data that would otherwise be useless. In the words of Jill Laise, the analytics manager at Annalect.com, a data-marketing subsidiary of the global marketing giant Omnicom Group, Inc. that spoke at a data marketing industry event, "Data is no good unless you do something with it."

Through a combination of possession, aggregation, and analyses, brokers make ownership claims over data that we produce. Chapter 5 of this book provides a deeper analysis of health data innovation and ownership. Regardless of the source of data, brokers often argue that through disclosure, data is made public and through data innovations, data is transformed into an asset that is owned by the innovator, the data broker. My concern here is how data that is produced through our everyday transactions are made "useful," engineered by data brokers to produce financial value and conform to a market logic.

Who Has Power over Our Data? Data Brokers Are Worse than the NSA

More than a year before Edward Snowden leaked information about the NSA's mass surveillance program to the press, in 2012 the US Senate Committee on Commerce, Science, and Transportation (Commerce Committee), the Federal Trade Commission (FTC), and the Government Accountability Office (GAO) were already preparing a full investigation into the data broker industry's mass surveillance of American consumers, and their possible violations of individuals' data privacy (Gidda 2013; Katz 2012; Federal Trade Commission 2012). Since the FTC is the primary regulatory agency in charge of consumer privacy and customer protection matters, there was growing concern among regulators about the burgeoning data brokerage sector's lack of transparency with regard to privacy and data security practices (Katz 2012). Many of the consumer privacy laws were written in earlier, pre-digital eras—though many have since been amended to address online privacy and data security concerns—privacy laws are only applicable by sector. There are no omnibus privacy laws that cover the data broker industry (Puente Cackley 2013, p. 7). Some twenty-eight legislative acts, dating back to the Privacy Act of 1974, contain some provision for personal information privacy yet it was obvious to the FTC that regulations were becoming increasingly inadequate to address the complexities of the data broker industry (Federal Trade Commission 2012). Before new regulations and practices could be proposed, however, there needed to be an investigation into how the data industry operates. This 2012 Congressional investigation revealed that the power the data brokerage industry holds over private information is stronger than that held by legislators.

In October 2012, Senator John D. (Jay) Rockefeller (D-WV), the chairman of the Senate Commerce Committee, sent letters to the nine largest data brokers in the USA requesting detailed information on how the companies acquire, compile, repackage, and sell data on millions of Americans. Rockefeller, a long-time advocate of consumer privacy, was gathering evidence in preparation for a Congressional hearing on the data broker industry set for 2013. Later that same year, the FTC, in collaboration with the Senate Commerce Committee and the GAO, began a parallel investigation of the data acquisition and data marketing industry and sent out an additional nine letters to data brokers requesting detailed information on how the industry collects and handles consumer data (Katz 2012). The Commerce Committee intended the hearing to investigate and to make public the data broker industry's secretive business practices, especially the sourcing, handling, and selling of the most private and sensitive details of consumers' lives for profit.

Three of the biggest companies that were subpoenaed—Acxiom, Experian, and Epsilon—refused to cooperate fully with the Committee and declined to provide details on their clients or the sources of the data that they hold (US Committee on Commerce, Science, and Transportation 2013, p. 10). Experian's senior vice president for government affairs, Tony Hadley, testified at the December 2013 Congressional hearing that "I can't tell you who our clients are…[t]hat's a proprietary list of ours. That's like our secret ingredient" (Tummarello 2013).

Hadley's refusal to cooperate with the Commerce Committee's request for more information was even more incredible since his refusal came on the heels of news in October 2013 that the company had been informed by the US Secret Service that the company had unwittingly sold personal identifying information records on more than 200 million US consumers to a Vietnamese identity theft ring in 2012 (Schwartz 2014; Krebs 2013). At the time, it was the company's largest breach in its history. Since then Experian has been subject to several more breaches, with another large one announced in October 2015. The corporation discovered that 15 million records of mobile communications company T-Mobile's customers (Experian conducts consumer credit checks for T-Mobile) had been illegally accessed since 2013, and hackers stole sensitive identity and financial data (Malik 2015). The data marketing and brokerage industry, as with many other industries when faced with regulatory scrutiny, maintains that the industry should self-regulate, albeit less aggressively than outsiders would, because they claim that as an industry they understand consumer informational privacy better than government (Urbanski 2015). As I show in the following chapter on privacy, self-regulation claims are usually just another way for the data broker industry to ensure that it is not cut off from its main resource: Consumer data.

During the 2013 hearings, Rockefeller stated that the data acquisition industry was "worse than the NSA" when it comes to the wholesale collection of private data on individuals (Tummarello 2013). Indeed, the government investigation and subsequent hearings were organized due to an increasing concern among both regulators and consumers about the processes of data collection and use by a largely unaccountable and opaque industry. Some of the results of the Senate committee hearings, as well as the GAO and FTC investigations, were embodied in the Data Broker Accountability and Transparency Act (the DATA Act) of 2014.[5] The DATA Act, sponsored by Rockefeller and Senator Edward (Ed) Markey (D-MA), outlined a regulatory regime that compels data brokers to be transparent in regard to the information they collect and how they profit from the sale of consumer data. The Act was immediately referred to the Commerce Committee, where, as of 2016, it still sits awaiting a legislative vote.

The Databased Society

Data collection and record keeping on citizens by governments and religious institutions is millennia old. Governments and empires, from the ancient Babylonians, Egyptians, and Romans through to the nation-state empires of modernity, conducted censuses to collect taxes and collected data on those living in conquered territories to control colonized or enslaved people (Scott 1999). The modern nation-state was built through the collection and standardization of population-derived data, instrumentalized for the "distribution of life chances across populations," or the management logic, the governmentality, of life (Foucault 2014; Spade 2011, p. 110; Dean 2012; Foucault 2008). Solove (2006) details how governmental data collected on residents increased exponentially during the nineteenth century when the collection of personal information became more richly detailed (and, for some, invasive and punitive) through population data collection. For instance, the first US Census, conducted in 1790, asked only four questions. By 1860, the census contained 142 questions. By the turn of the twentieth century, citizens began to push back on the large number and nature of the census questions (Solove 2006, pp. 13–14). The concomitant rise of bureaucratic agencies in the USA during the twentieth century necessitated richer and more detailed information, as well as improved systems to collect, store, organize, and analyze these increasingly huge amounts of data (Scott 1999).

One of the earliest *industries* to collect, secure, and disclose individuals' personal information, including health data, was insurers and actuaries. In fact, the insurance industry is one of the first among private enterprise to collect personal information on a mass scale and, through analytics, make biologically derived data adhere to a market logic, rather than a logic of population management and control (Scott 1999; Foucault 1990). The insurers of the Atlantic slave trade, for instance, those American companies that paid out money to investors when a slave ship they owned capsized or when enslaved people did not survive the Middle Passage, collected detailed health and other pertinent information on the human cargo. Data was collected about the individual children, women, and men who had been kidnapped and sold into slavery. The health insurer Aetna Inc. was sued in 2002, along with several other insurance companies, for profiting off nineteenth-century slavery. Aetna's predecessor company sold thousands of life insurance policies to slave owners in the case that their slaves died of natural causes; of course, many of those deaths were not natural in the least (Groark 2002). Vivian Zelizer describes another corner of the insurance industry: child life insurance. In her account of the burgeoning (and highly controversial at the time) sector during the nineteenth century, Zelizer explains that company salesmen collected data on children within the households of policy holders—usually poor and working-class parents who depended on the financial value of their children through the children's labor power (and thus, considered good "prospects" by the insurance industry)—during their weekly visits to collect premiums (Zelizer 1981). Part of that weekly data collection included the current state of the insured children's health, and an accounting of the number of children, in case a child died.

The nineteenth century was also an era when companies began collecting financial information, especially on the credit-worthiness of customers. The earliest insurers also formed during this time, collecting information such as debts owed or outstanding, and sharing this information among retailers on a local level. In an Experian account of its corporate history, the company claims that part of its origins can be traced back to a small association of innkeepers, retailers, and tradespeople, *The Society of Guardians for the Protection of Tradesmen Against Swindlers, Sharpers and Other Fraudulent Persons*, formed in 1826 in Manchester, England. The Society gathered information on known persons who failed to pay their bills or committed fraud against the Society's associates, and published its findings in a monthly circular distributed to members. In recognition that the gathered information was, in large part, based on gossip and hearsay, the Society created a "data accuracy officer" to vet collected information for inaccuracies (Watson 2013, pp. 2–3).

In the twentieth century, the credit industry expanded exponentially with the attendant rise of computing power, software, and database engineering, especially during the 1980s. Simultaneously, the credit and finance industries were undergoing mass deregulation, which opened up consumer credit for middle-to-low income Americans. In the process, the credit risk industry moved the credit history information held on 90 percent of Americans from three-by-five index cards in massive warehouses to integrated databases enabling data brokers to efficiently and expeditiously collect, store, mine, and package complex information from diverse sources (Solove 2006). This move of data from paper to the digital changed not only the storage of data, but also what *kind* of data could be stored and what kind of analysis could be done on it. Digital media scholars Viktor Mayer-Schönberger and Kenneth Cukier use the term "datafication" to name this partnering of computing power with the mass collection of information that is "recorded, analyzed, and reorganized." Datafication means the ability to transform phenomena into a quantifiable format (Mayer-Schönberger and Cukier 2012, p. 77). A societal logic that sees value in the measurement, quantification and categorization of phenomena, everything from the radiation output of quasars to the number of clicks on a website, is subjected to datafication.

The data brokerage industry grew out of two sectors: credit reporting and data marketing. Credit reporting companies are able to collect massive amounts of data on consumers when they seek lines of credit: mortgages, consumer and personal loans, credit cards, and other debit instruments that require creditors to investigate the creditworthiness and risks associated with extending credit to an individual consumer. Similarly, marketing companies also collect data. These data services that they provide constitutes what I contend contributes to the "databased society," a culture that produces economic value based on the datafication of human life. Our data images are distributed across databases and are summoned by marketing entities to produce value for those who possess these data.

Marketing segmentation is part of the overall trend that has moved mass marketing to target marketing, which is increasingly fueled by data analytics and big data. Market segmentation is a method of dividing an entire market into subsets of consumers, based on commonly shared characteristics such as household income and financial resources, geographic location, family size, inferred psychological make-up and cultural attitudes (also known within the industry as "psychographics"), and demographics such as age or gender. The technique of dividing heterogeneous markets into homogeneous clusters of individuals with similar desires and needs, inferred by market research, has transformed not only how goods and services are sold and consumed, but also virtually all communications with the public (Doyle 2011).

Marketing data analytics that segment individuals into particular profiles, especially via psychographics and lifestyle attributes, is not limited to marketing alone; segmentation studies are used in everything from electoral politics to public health research (Nielsen 2012; Luntz 2007; Grier and Bryant 2005; Slater and Flora 1991). Turow (2010) argues that marketing segmentation is one of the driving forces behind the logic of a "databased" society; big data and marketing were made for each other:

> The industrial logic leads [marketing executives] to work toward a century in which databases rule. It is a world where biometric data recognition provides executives with a secure sense of who the entering consumer is; where customizations in programming, product offerings and price discounts take place instantly based on customer history and niche identification; and where the entire process reinforces the consumer in the relationship while adding the information about the encounter to the dataset so that the next encounter will be more profitable. (Turow 2010, p. 6934)

The segmentation of people into marketing categories for targeted and fine-grained communications arose in the 1960s as a marketing innovation and has, in part, driven the collapse of the imaginary line between "citizen" and "consumer." Market segmentation is the backbone of database marketing, and comprises the core business of many data brokers. Significantly, as computational power has increased exponentially, the data analytics that comprise marketing segmentation in the age of big data is nothing short of what media theorist John Cheney-Lippold calls "algorithmic identity," where our online and offline behaviors are collated by marketers and where algorithmic inferences "allow a shift to a more flexible and functional definition of the category, one that de-essentializes [identity] from its corporeal and societal forms and determinations while it also re-essentializes [identity] as a statistically related, largely market research-driven category" (2011, p. 170. My addition in brackets). In the example that Cheney-Lippold provides, the embodied and societal category of a particular gender is decoupled from the individual person who identifies with a particular gender, and redeployed into a free-floating marketing category of "male" or "female" (marketing logic is often binary—gender, race and class categories that defy facile categorization are rendered invisible) that has particular habits, desires, and of course, predictable consumption behaviors that can be targeted with specific marketing messages.

Experian Marketing Services, the marketing arm of the credit bureau Experian plc that sold my consumer profile to list broker ALC, grew out of a series of mergers and acquisitions. Bain Capital brokered the first merger between the American credit bureau TRW Information Services and the UK credit scoring company CCN, creating the new company dubbed "Experian" (Watson 2013, pp. 15–17). It is through this series of mergers and demergers, that Experian plc became an Irish company with its global headquarters in Nottingham, United Kingdom.[6] In its promotional materials Experian claims that its four core business operations include decision analytics, credit services, consumer services and marketing services (Experian plc 2016).

One of Experian's market segmentation products is Mosaic USA (the Mosaic platform is also customized for fifteen other countries), and the product's promotional brochure states that the seventy-one segments available through the Mosaic platform are derived from consumer data on 116 million US households. Globally, the platform holds data on two billion individuals (Experian Marketing Services 2016, p. 5). Experian claims that the Mosaic product builds these profiles from more than 300 separate data "attributes," or sources and does not delineate further what the data are or how they were aggregated. This is all Experian's "secret sauce." What are not so secret are the categories of how the lives of people are sliced up and made into flat, data images—marketers' stereotypes of the complex lives of millions of strangers. Households are hierarchically labeled from those in the highest income brackets "A—Power Elite" to the bottom economic rung "S—Economic Challenges," and the subcategories further divide these 116 million households into slots based on data analytics and a lot of marketing story-telling embellishments. The subcategories or segments are given such titles as "American Royalty," "Platinum Prosperity," and "Aspirational Fusions—Dare to Dream," or "Families in Motion—Diapers and Debit Cards" (Experian Marketing Services 2016, pp. 7–8).

What is striking in reading these categories is that despite the (presumably) highly sophisticated algorithmic analyses that went into mining the large amounts of data to refine it into marketing meaningful segments, the resulting categories read as trite and glib which simply recapitulate well-worn racial, gender and class biases. One of the ways that these biases are displayed is in the stock photos used to illustrate some of the categories. Each photograph depicts models that are white, appear to be healthy, well-dressed and holding objects—smart phones, shopping bags, and paper cups of coffee—that mark their class status. The one model of color, an African-American girl of about six years of age, is playfully held in the arms of a smiling white man, with a white woman and another white girl, blurred in the background, meant to imply that this is a family made through transracial adoption, again another indicator of class status. The Mosaic brochure does not visually depict any of the other segmentation categories, such as "Red, White and Bluegrass," "Modest Metro Means," "Urban Survivors," or "Small Town Shallow Pockets," or any number of the working class and poor, older generational, racially inferred categories. Presumably, these are not "good prospects" for many marketers that may use the Experian product and indicate that the "algorithmic identities" constructed by Mosaic are limited to racialized and classed notions of consumers. These algorithmic identities become the instruments of "data phrenology" for the databased society.

Private health data is buried within these various marketing categories, since not only does Experian collect search and purchasing data behaviors that we transact both online and offline, including searches on diseases or symptoms and purchases of health services, the company offers another data product, Experian Health, through which the broker collects health and medical data, in a similar way that it collects data through its credit risk platforms used by creditors. While of course these data will be de-identified and considered HIPAA-compliant, it is certainly possible that these Experian Health-derived data will be aggregated into various data assets, including the Mosaic product. Your detective suspects that the marketing baby, at least parts of its body, may reside in one of the Mosaic categories and this is a lead that should be investigated further. Through the data that Experian collects on us through our online and offline behaviors, they are able to analyze and make inferences about us, and sell these inferences to other marketers. This wholesale collection of personal data remains almost entirely invisible to us because most data brokers do not have direct contact with consumers, but rather contract with "consumer facing" businesses, from large multinational retailers to small non-profits and which directly collect data on us.

How is it that there is an industry, an industry that most of us have never heard of, that is so powerful that it can remain behind a curtain of secrecy and refuse to cooperate with government when subpoenaed to do so? The industry is able to do this, I contend, at least in part, because they claim ownership over our data. They are able to make these ownership claims in two very important ways. The first way is that data comes to "rest" or "land" into their database warehouses through either actively sourcing data or by passively collecting data through data contracts with clients. It is through the second way that brokers take ownership over our data that is even stronger than mere possession; after all, data at rest is dead data. Brokers argue that by "adding value" to data through analyzing it, processing it, de-identifying it, and creating new instruments or data products out of "raw" data, brokers firm up their ownership claims. A common refrain in the industry is that data is the "new oil" and brokers are the "processors" that refine it and make it into "products." Innovation equals ownership.

Furthermore, data companies, such as Experian, are able to analyze and make inferences about us and sell these inferences to other marketers. By making proprietary claims and remaining secretive about their data sources as well as about how they build their data assets, are all ways that they maintain their power. In Chapters 4 and 5, I develop how these ownership claims are made with health data. The power that data brokers wield over personal data comes from their ownership claims through possession and innovation, and ultimately, through our dispossession of our data.

Notes

1. Most data brokers will go to pains explaining that customers do "consent" to the massive data collection that occurs, primarily through the "opt in" agreements placed before a customer during a transaction. As Fuchs (2014) and others have shown, many of these are 16 pages or longer, and the consent clause is usually buried within complex text, so while ostensibly a company like Experian can claim that they have a customer's consent, many consumers believe that this is a fallacy.
2. See Experian Marketing Services' patent holdings in the United States Patent and Trademark Office's database: http://www.uspto.gov/patent.
3. Tanner details how Caesars Palace collects transactional, behavioral and other types of data, including location data, on its patrons that are enrolled in its Total Rewards program and its Total Rewards credit card. Through Caesars's credit card, the casino is able to track patrons' transactional behavior in rival casinos, as well as other retailers and service providers.
4. Experian Health is a data and software platform, and part of Experian's business services: http://www.experian.com/healthcare/experian-healthcare.html.
5. The Data Broker Accountability and Transparency Act is not to be confused with the Digital Accountability and Transparency Act of 2014 (DATA Act) that called for more rigorous accountability in regards to the information concerning government expenditures and budgetary transparency. The Digital Accountability and Transparency Act was signed into law on May 9, 2014.
6. As of January 2016, Experian's corporate website lists that it employs 17,000 people in 38 countries. Previously, in 2014, the company claimed to have offices in 40 countries (Experian plc 2016).

References

Acxiom Corporation. 2015a. *About Acxiom*. Acxiom. Accessed January 9, 2016. http://www.acxiom.com/about-acxiom.

———. 2015b. "Acxiom Annual Report 2015." Annual Report to Shareholders; Securities and Exchange Commission (SEC) filings SEC FORM 10-K. Little Rock, AR: Acxiom.

American List Counsel Inc. 2015. "Mh2 PrecisionBase Ailment Masterfile." Business website. *Data Cards*. http://datacards.alc.com/market;jsessionid=F308D87AC06243ACD2F2A7F2421C679A?page=research/datacard&id=268734.

Angwin, Julia. 2015. *Dragnet Nation: A Quest for Privacy, Security, and Freedom in a World of Relentless Surveillance*. New York: St. Martin's Griffin.

Barocas, Solon, and Helen Nissenbaum. 2014. "Big Data's End Run Around Procedural Privacy Protections." *Communications of the ACM* 57 (11): 31–33.

Cheney-Lippold, John. 2011. "A New Algorithmic Identity: Soft Biopolitics and the Modulation of Control." *Theory, Culture & Society* 28 (6): 164–81.

Corrin, Amber. 2015. "TSA Pulls Back on Big-Data PreCheck Expansion." *Federal Times*, February 16. Accessed January 9, 2016. http://www.federaltimes.com/story/government/dhs/programs/2015/02/16/tsa-pulls-back-on-big-data-precheck-expansion/23513781.

Dean, Mitchell. 2012. "The Signature of Power." *Journal of Political Power* 5 (1): 101–17.

Doyle, Charles. 2011. *A Dictionary of Marketing*. 3rd ed. Oxford: Oxford University Press.

Experian Marketing Services. 2016. *Mosaic® USA: The Consumer Classification Solution for Consistent Cross-Channel Marketing*. Experian Marketing Services, October. Accessed January 9, 2016. http://www.experian.com/assets/marketing-services/brochures/mosaic-brochure-october-2014.pdf.

Experian plc. "Experian Plc About Us." Promotional website. Our Four Business Lines, 2016. https://www.experianplc.com/about-us/.

Federal Trade Commission. 2012. *Protecting Consumer Privacy in an Era of Rapid Change: Recommendations for Businesses and Policymakers*. Washington, DC: Federal Trade Commission. https://www.ftc.gov/reports/protecting-consumer-privacy-era-rapid-change-recommendations-businesses-policymakers.

———. 2014. *Data Brokers: Call for Transparency and Accountability*. Washington, DC: Federal Trade Commission. https://www.ftc.gov/system/files/documents/reports/data-brokers-call-transparency-accountability-report-federal-trade-commission-may-2014/140527databrokerreport.pdf.

Foucault, Michel. 1990. *The History of Sexuality: Volume I*. Translated by Robert Hurley. New York: Pantheon.

———. 2008. *The Birth of Biopolitics: Lectures at the Collège de France, 1978–79*. Translated by Graham Burchell and edited by Michel Senellart. New York: Palgrave Macmillian.

———. 2014. *On the Government of the Living: Lectures at the Collège de France, 1979-1980*. Translated by Graham Burchell and edited by Michel Senellart. New York: Palgrave Macmillian.

Fuchs, Christian. 2014. *Social Media: A Critical Introduction*. London: Sage.

Gidda, Mirren. 2013. "Edward Snowden and the NSA Files: Timeline." *Guardian*, August 21. Accessed January 9, 2016. http://www.theguardian.com/world/2013/jun/23/edward-snowden-nsa-files-timeline.

Grier, Sonya, and Carol A. Bryant. 2005. "Social Marketing in Public Health." *Annual Review of Public Health* 26: 319–35.

Groark, Virginia. 2002. "Slave Policies." *New York Times*, May 5. Accessed January 9, 2016. http://www.nytimes.com/2002/05/05/nyregion/slave-policies.html.

Katz, Mitchell J. 2012. *FTC to Study Data Broker Industry's Collection and Use of Consumer Data*. Federal Trade Commission. Accessed January 9, 2016. https://www.ftc.gov/news-events/press-releases/2012/12/ftc-study-data-broker-industrys-collection-use-consumer-data.

Krebs, Brian. 2013. "Experian Sold Consumer Data to ID Theft Service." *KrebsonSecurity*, October 20. Accessed January 9, 2016. http://krebsonsecurity.com/2013/10/experian-sold-consumer-data-to-id-theft-service/.

Luntz, Frank. 2007. *Words That Work: It's Not What You Say, It's What People Hear*. New York: Hyperion.

Magill-Cook, Lori. 2015a. "Write-Ups on Experian's Newborn Network Database," August 4.

———. 2015b. "The New Parent Market Is Growing (and Spending)," December 5.

Malik, Om. 2015. "Why Companies Won't Learn From the T-Mobile/Experian Hack." *New Yorker*, October 6. Accessed January 9, 2016. http://www.newyorker.com/business/currency/why-companies-wont-learn-from-the-t-mobileexperian-hack.

Mayer-Schönberger, Viktor, and Kenneth Cukier. 2012. *Big Data: A Revolution That Transforms How We Work, Live, and Think*. Boston, MA: Houghton Mifflin Harcourt.

Nielsen, Rasmus Kleis. 2012. *Ground Wars: Personalized Communication in Political Campaigns*. Princeton, NJ: Princeton University Press.

Puente Cackley, Alicia. 2013. *Information Resellers: Consumer Privacy Framework Needs to Reflect Changes in Technology and the Marketplace*. GAO-13-663. Washington, DC: Government Accountability Office.

Samilton, Tracy. 2015. "Being a Loyal Auto Insurance Customer Can Cost You." *NPR.com*, May 8. Accessed January 9, 2016. http://www.npr.org/2015/05/08/403598235/being-a-loyal-auto-insurance-customer-can-cost-you.

Schwartz, Matthew J. 2014. "Experian ID Theft Exposed 200M Consumer Records." *Information Week's Dark Reading*, March 11. Accessed January 9, 2016. http://www.darkreading.com/attacks-and-breaches/experian-id-theft-exposed-200m-consumer-records/d/d-id/1127640.

Scott, James C. 1999. *Seeing Like a State: How Certain Schemes to Improve the Human Condition Have Failed*. New Haven, CT: Yale University Press.

Sheer, Robert, and Sara Beladi. 2015. *They Know Everything About You: How Data-Collecting Corporations and Snooping Government Agencies Are Destroying Democracy*. New York: Nation Books.

Singer, Natasha. 2012. "You for Sale: Mapping, and Sharing, the Consumer Genome." *New York Times*, June 17, sec. Technology, BU1.

Slater, M. D., and J. A. Flora. 1991. "Health Lifestyles: Audience Segmentation Analysis for Public Health Interventions." *Health Education Quarterly* 18 (2): 221–33.

Solove, Daniel J. 2006. *The Digital Person: Technology and Privacy in the Information Age*. New York: New York University Press.

Spade, Dean. 2011. *Normal Life: Administrative Violence, Critical Trans Politics and the Limits of the Law*. Brooklyn, NY: South End Press.

Steel, Emily. 2013a. "Companies Scramble for Consumer Data." *Financial Times*, June 12, sec. Media. http://www.ft.com/intl/cms/s/0/f0b6edc0-d342-11e2-b3ff-00144feab7de.html#axzz3hUIXlcqc.

———. 2013b. "Financial Worth of Data Comes in at Under a Penny a Piece." *Financial Times*, June 12, New York edition, sec. FT.com. http://www.ft.com/intl/cms/s/0/3cb056c6-d343-11e2-b3ff-00144feab7de.html#axzz3nu3UQteG.

Tanner, Adam. 2014. *What Stays in Vegas: The World of Personal Data, Lifeblood of Big Business and the End of Privacy as We Know It*. New York: PublicAffairs, Perseus.

Tummarello, Kate. 2013. "Rockefeller: 'Data Brokers' Worse than NSA Spying." *Hill*, December 18. Accessed January 10, 2016. http://thehill.com/policy/technology/193576-rockefeller-data-brokers-worse-than-nsa-spying.

Turow, Joseph. 2010. "Segment-Making and Society-Making Media: What Is a Good Balance?" *The Harmony of Civilization and Prosperity for All: Selected Papers of Beijing Forum (2004–2008)* 2 (5): 6928–36.

Urbanski, Al. 2015. "Redefining Data Privacy." *DM News*, May 1. Accessed January 10, 2016. http://www.dmnews.com/dataanalytics/redefining-data-privacy/article/410810.

US Committee on Commerce, Science, and Transportation. 2013. *A Review of the Data Broker Industry: Collection, Use, and Sale of Consumer Data for Marketing Purposes*. Washington, DC: Office of Oversight and Investigations. http://www.commerce.senate.gov/public/?a=Files.Serve&File_id=0d2b3642-6221-4888-a631-08f2f255b577.

Watson, Nigel. "A Brief History of Experian: Our Story." Dublin: Experian plc, September 2013. https://www.experianplc.com/media/1323/8151-exp-experian-history-book_abridged_final.pdf.

Zelizer, Viviana A. 1981. "The Price and Value of Children: The Case of Children's Insurance." *American Journal of Sociology* 86 (5): 1036–56.

CHAPTER 3

Privacy and Data Phantoms

The Biopolitics of Phantom Data

As patients we produce data in excessive amounts, so much so it has been described as a flood, a data deluge that statistical science has yet to develop sufficient methods to probe (Sagoff 2012, p. 71; Merchant 2008; Balasanov 2015). Our bodies, in fact, are founts of data, which is made "useful" not only for individual patient care, but for all sorts of industries. Our lungs, hearts, uteri, ovaries, spermatozoa, oocytes, spleens, colons, umbilical cords, urine, blood, kidneys, anuses, livers, feces, brains, cells, and DNA, as well as the DNA of other species that we carry within and on us—like bacteria or cancers—are photographed, scanned, probed, excised, measured, and quantified, and thus transformed into data. This fleshy data increasingly ends up in databases stored in data warehouses, separated from the bodies that produced it. Poet Daniel Borzutzky describes this dematerialization of embodied data in his poem *The Data Harbor*:

> She sends my body through the fax machine because I contain vital information that might make or break the bureaucrats on the other end, but when I arrive through the wires I am stored in a box and put in a basement and a few months later the basement floods and I am stuck forever amid boxes of flooded data. (2015, p. 69)

Is there anything more intimate than the living materials that make us, that sustain our bodies or that kill us? What could be a more fraught, and a more potent, symbol of the conditions of the Age of Big Data than the

M.F.E. Ebeling, *Healthcare and Big Data*,
DOI 10.1057/978-1-137-50221-6_3

fact that pieces of us live digital lives outside of our bodies? Those pieces are maintained and optimized to produce value—primarily financial and marketing value—through clicks and keystrokes done by strangers, many of whom have never met us and never will, and who would never have such intimate access to our bodies under other circumstances.

The data that our bodies produce can have a direct impact on our health: A doctor collects a tissue sample; it is analyzed and transformed into data that can tell the doctor whether or not the sample is cancerous; and that information will direct the treatment of an individual patient. More often, however, our data are put to work not for our direct benefit, but for the benefit of others. Public health researchers use large datasets of outpatient surgery records from hospitals, for instance, to study the effectiveness of certain procedures that potentially could benefit not just one, but thousands of patients. Patients with rare or debilitating diseases often weigh the balance between keeping their health status private against sharing their data in open online forums, such as Patientslikeme.com, in exchange for medical researchers' promise that their data would benefit others similarly diagnosed (Ali et al. 2015). For these patient advocates, it does not matter that the website is a commercial one, a data platform that benefits from pharmaceutical and medical industry investments as well as partnerships with health research non-profits; they give their data freely knowing that it could be commercialized. The potential risks to their privacy is worth the possible benefits to their health and well-being, and it could help other patients as well (Professional Services Close-Up 2014).

I began this book with the birth story of my data phantom—my marketing baby—a birth that took place not in the clinic but in a data broker's database. The book itself was born out of betrayal and violation: I had an expectation of privacy in my doctor's office, an expectation that many of us may have. But why? How did I come to believe that the information that was collected from my body or about my health and disclosed in my doctor's office would not be shared with anyone else outside of the context of healthcare provision? How was my sense of privacy stretched and breached by the collection and commodification of my health data?

Perhaps it is because as our vitality is being digitized, we increasingly live with a seeming contradiction. Many of us have a desire to keep certain things about us and our lives private; we often believe that this desire is inherent in the human condition and central to human dignity, at least in the abstract. Yet, we also live with the knowledge that everything we do and say is often being tracked, watched, recorded, and gathered, especially digitally. Some of us believe that if we are doing nothing wrong, then we have nothing to worry about. But many of us—those who are members of historically marginalized groups, including people with disabilities, migrants, racial, gender and sexual minorities—have never had an expectation of privacy, indeed, quite the opposite. Many of us live with the trauma and fear of never having a right to privacy whatsoever. In her extraordinary book *Private Bodies, Public Texts*, bio-ethicist and legal scholar Karla Holloway notes that within the social, political, and economic contexts of privacy, expectations are conditional: "As human as the right to privacy may seem, it has a public history that absolutely renders it a socially selective privilege" (Holloway 2011, p. 7).

You may have noticed that things have changed over the years, although the changes become imperceptible as we form them into habits—at some point, some of us swapped out a paper journal to divulge our most secretive thoughts before we go to sleep for online Facebook disclosures without bothering to change our privacy settings (as if that would make a difference anyhow). We disclose some of our most intimate and sensitive information in very open and public ways not only online but offline as well. For some of us, as long as we have control over the disclosure context, this can be empowering. In response to recent legislative encroachment on women's reproductive rights, some women who have had an abortion are telling their "abortion stories" online to undermine the social stigma of terminating a pregnancy and to emphasize that such a choice, while not an easy one, is ultimately a private one.[1] Women who make their abortion stories public, ultimately wrest control over their story by choosing to make their private decision a political, *public* act (Bahadur 2015).[2] The key here is that women who tell their abortion stories online are in control of the context of disclosure. What I hope to demonstrate throughout this chapter is that in most cases in which health data is collected and disclosed, patients not only do not control the context, they have no way of knowing the complexity of the data networks that disclosures are made within, to whom those disclosures are made and or what is made of those disclosures.

We are often less aware of offline disclosures, since these come in the form of a credit card swipe or a PIN entered into an ATM. Yet, so long as our behavior is in some way digitized, information on every detail of our lives is being disclosed somewhere, by someone. Sometimes that someone is us, sometimes it is a stranger, but it always involves an algorithm and a database. And there is little that we can do about it.

We are often outraged when we learn that "our privacy" has been breached, especially if that breach is done by those who have some kind of power over our lives, such as the police, a bank, or the government. Yet, in what seems to be a direct contradiction to our indignation, we go through our daily routines, knowing full well that everything we do online, on our phones, out in public (especially in ostensibly "public spaces" enclosed by commerce) is being tracked, and data on every transaction we make is being collected.

In their book *Obfuscation*, a little volume filled with practical strategies to flummox Big Data, privacy scholars Finn Brunton and Helen Nissenbaum incisively sum up the daily contradictions of privacy and "information asymmetry":

> We can see a surveillance camera mounted on a streetlight, or concealed in a dome of mirrored glass on the ceiling of a hallway, and we know that we are being recorded. We know that we don't know whether the recording is being transmitted only on the site or ... streamed over the Internet ... [w]e don't know if the footage is being run through facial-recognition software ... or if the time code can be correlated with a credit-card purchase ... to connect our image with our identity—in fact, unless we are personally involved with privacy activism or security engineering, we don't know that we don't know that. ... And that is merely one CCTV camera ... [m]ultiply this by making a credit-card purchase, signing up for an email list, downloading a smartphone app ("This app requires access to your contacts"? "Sure!"), giving a postal code or a birthday or a [sic] identification number in response to a reasonable and legitimate request, and on and on through the day and around the world. (Brunton and Nissenbaum 2015, loc 978)

Often, we consider certain categories of data particularly sacrosanct, such as information about our health or family, thinking that these data warrant extra protection from disclosure. While there is legislative recognition that certain data or groups of people require extra privacy protections, evidenced in laws such as the Health Insurance Portability and Accountability Act (HIPAA) (legislation that I discuss at greater length in Chapter 4) and the Children's Online Privacy Protection Act (COPPA), most laws have failed to keep up with innovations in digital technologies and data collection practices. In an effort to stem the flow of commercial data away from citizens and into the hands of corporations, in March 2015, the Obama administration released a draft of the Consumer Privacy Bill of Rights. Upon its release, however, many privacy rights observers noted that the draft bill lacked any legislative teeth, possibly preempted established state privacy laws, and did nothing to prevent sensitive data (such as patient health information) from being sold to marketers.

The public often expresses greater outrage when particular types of data, especially sensitive data related to health, are exposed—except when we make these unfortunate disclosures through our own behavior, in which case we often castigate ourselves (we know better than to give a stranger our private data!). Several data services industries, in particular the database marketing and data brokerage industries, actively lobby against privacy regulations, as industrial spokespeople often argue that they are best suited to regulate themselves. In the face of such asymmetrical power over the privacy of data, we seem to be resigned to the fact that we are powerless when it comes to protecting our informational privacy, and helpless to prevent how our data are used in ways that can potentially harm us (Turow et al. 2015).

Surely some of us have experienced something like what happened to Claudia. Living in a small northeastern US town, she told me in an interview that she often frequented a retail drug store to purchase toiletries and to have the occasional prescription filled. Claudia also used a customer loyalty card, given to her by the drug store in exchange for her name, address, phone number, and (when swiped) information on her purchases. She had the card swiped at checkout for most purchases, including prescriptions. For a time, she noticed that her receipts offered coupons for "diabetes-related" products, such as discounts on needles and at-home glucose monitors. Claudia found this curious since she thought that neither her prescriptions nor the items that she occasionally purchased indicated that she had diabetes. Yet, the drug store's data image of her reflected a diagnosis: diabetes. In fact, during the time that Claudia started to notice that the drug store's database had diagnosed her, she also received phone calls from charities fundraising for diabetes research. Somehow, her data image leaked out from the drug store's database and into the hands of at least one charity. Claudia never was able to discern how the drug store determined that she "had" diabetes and at some point, she noticed that the diabetes-related coupon offers and phone calls ceased as mysteriously as they had begun.

What happened to Claudia happened to me as well, and often happens to others in this Age of Big Data. We hand over personal information about ourselves, either consenting to it knowingly or not, only to be haunted by that data when it comes back to us in some sort of phantom data-marketing image of ourselves. Even when we consciously attempt to render ourselves invisible to Big Data by opting out, the system eyes us suspiciously, as was the case for sociologist Janet Vertesi. When she became pregnant, she went to extreme efforts to hide her pregnancy from digital media and from data brokers, by phoning friends and family with her news, by not searching online for pregnancy-related information or products, by paying for everything in cash. In her experiment, she found that her data image was one of a criminal because Big Data could not index her behavior; she was illegible as a consumer (Vertesi 2014). Sometimes we might laugh it off as an incongruous ghostly mirage, but there are other times, when perhaps we are hurting, vulnerable, or trying to hold on to our lives as we are dying of cancer or losing a loved one, when a data ghost comes knocking at our doors, wanting to be let in to further hurt and traumatize us (Pearce 2014).[3] While my focus here is on aggregation and commodification of personal health data by commercial interests, there are numerous contexts in which such bodily data can harm us. For example, the collection and use of biological data by the state or even by insurers, say when blood and DNA samples are collected from immigration applicants or incarcerated youth, can have huge and traumatic implications for the person's life (Duster 2003).

Lively Data and Vaporized Privacy Rights

What are we to make of our phantom data? How can we prevent being haunted and traumatized by our data, data that is reanimated by marketing and algorithms, takes on a life of its own, and stomps clumsily back into our lives? How did our privacy vanish? Is this disappearance related to dead-cum-lively data or did we ever have a right to privacy in the first place?

While the concept of privacy can be hard to define—what one person might consider "private" may not be considered so by others—and as privacy values and behaviors are culturally and contextually dependent, defining "privacy" becomes very difficult indeed (Acquisti *et al.* 2015, p. 513). Some privacy scholars argue that privacy means everything and nothing at all, and that while it might seem to be a culturally specific value, it is a principle that is shared universally across cultures and historic periods—and often reflects overarching ideological commitments of a society. For some privacy scholars, activists, and regulators, especially those working in health and medicine, privacy pertains to the collection, storage, and use of personal information or data that is individually identifiable (Nass *et al.* 2009, p. 16). Much of the US privacy legislation passed since the mid-twentieth century has defined privacy as the protection of individual facts about a person from being exposed to public scrutiny without their consent, or the protection of individuals from certain intrusions into what is considered a private space. However, many people have a more expansive notion of privacy than these laws provide. Most people have a sense of what is "private," even if what is considered to be private changes across cultures, epochs, and even people who share a culture (Solove 2006, pp. 481–482). A sense of privacy may relate to who may have access to our bodies, thoughts, behaviors, or relationships, both intimate and otherwise. More so, how privacy is defined can profoundly disadvantage certain groups. For example, calling salary information private can mask pay inequality between men and women, calling home life "private" can perpetuate familial violence by keeping it "in the family," and even calling healthcare experiences private can hide implicit bias and racial and gender discrimination in healthcare settings. In cases of asymmetrical power, the struggle to make something public or to keep it secret is a political one (Benhabib 2007, p. 94). Yet, the implications of privacy can deeply harm those who are disempowered when privacy serves the interests of the powerful. Media scholar Christian Fuchs notes this when considering how privacy has advantaged the wealthy elite and disadvantaged those who do not enjoy the same privacy rights. For example, the wealthy are often able to maintain offshore bank accounts in countries that keep these secret from tax bureaus (Fuchs 2014). In the contemporary USA, privacy's legal definitions often stem from the ideological concepts of the liberal self and the autonomous subject (Cohen 2013). The contemporary notion that individuals should enjoy privacy can be traced to nineteenth-century liberal Enlightenment ideology, which is foundational to US law (Fuchs 2014, p. 156). Fundamental to the liberal ideal of privacy is a core concern with individual autonomy; for an individual to be independent, especially in relation to government power, she or he must be imbued legally with certain inalienable rights, including the right to conceal or disclose personal information. In their definitive 1890 article "The Right of Privacy," Samuel Warren and Louis Brandeis trace the evolution of individual rights from common law, especially the rights to life and property, to the legal recognition of "corporeal property" and the incorporeal properties and rights issuing from the "legal" possession of one's own body, such as artistic expression, ideas, and inventions, thus linking the right to privacy to the right of intellectual property. They argued that the approach of the twentieth century required that "the right to be left alone" be codified, as the era saw rapid changes in new media technologies capable of capturing an "essence" of an individual, including descriptive photography and mass media. They also argued that intangibles, such as thoughts, emotions, and personal characteristics, should be considered an individual's "property" and thus enjoy a right to privacy, "a right to one's personality" (Warren and Brandeis 1890, p. 205). Holloway points to the class, race, and gender positionality of Warren and Brandeis, and argues that for them, the right to privacy was connected to an "inviolate personhood" in which privacy was an "intimate aspect of identity" inseparable from the body (2011, p. 28). She notes that such a perspective on privacy could only come from White, male, upper class subjects. After all, African Americans have historically been denied this bodily "inviolate personhood" both under slavery and afterwards, a denial legally codified just a few years after Warren and Brandeis's 1890 article in *Plessy v. Ferguson's* 1896 "separate but equal" doctrine (2011, pp. 27–30). Certainly many of the social justice and identity movements that arose in the twentieth and twenty-first centuries—from the Civil Rights Movement to Reproductive Rights to Stonewall to the Dreamers—were, in part, concerned with a struggle over the right to "inviolate personhood."

Legal scholar Julie Cohen argues that considering the current conditions of informational privacy, we should understand ourselves to be "postliberal subjects." We are not autonomous individuals living on islands of privacy (and we never were), but rather we are situated in messy, complex social relationships that co-produce our emergent subjectivities (Cohen 2013, p. 1910). So too, ideas, beliefs, and legislation about what constitutes the distinction between public space and private domains in Western cultural contexts are fluid, and these distinctions have in some ways collapsed through digital media and communication technologies. Some see this collapse as mundane and harmless, and others see it as dangerous and traumatic. If I speak on my smartphone on the bus, I don't expect my conversation to be private. However, if on the same bus ride, I use my smartphone to browse the Internet for information about a high blood pressure diagnosis, I might assume or at least hope that my search history is private (unless another rider looks over my shoulder). But this is a completely unreasonable assumption on my part since, as I described in Chapter 2, virtually all of my online and offline behaviors are being captured and shared digitally. As Josh Sims, a bioinformatics engineer, described it to me during an interview, data privacy expectations and legislation simply cannot keep up with the algorithms.

Since the 1973 Federal report on privacy and information technologies that outlined the Fair Information Practice Principles (FIPPS) framework, US law has considered informational privacy through two mechanisms: consent and anonymization (Barocas and Nissenbaum 2014, p. 32). Consent here entails that we, as data subjects, understand that our data is being collected, analyzed, and commodified, and that we give our permission for this to happen. Anonymization means that as part of consent process, we also consent to this data collection as long as it will be decoupled from us and de-identified—our information is not supposed to be able to come back to haunt us. Here is one of the legal fictions of big data and database marketing: The *de jure* legal rule stands in stark contrast with the daily *de facto* data hauntings.

Social media scholar danah boyd points out that for quite a long time we have attempted to control the information that may be disclosed about us, instead of trying to control the social context of disclosure (Marwick and boyd 2014; boyd 2014). She notes that younger generations that have grown up with the Internet understand this, while legislators are trying to catch up with constantly changing information technologies. Context is everything. Just as we are social beings without "autonomous, precultural cores," we are selves entangled within social, cultural, and political contexts that are in flux, particularly online. In this world, privacy cannot be a "fixed condition," but should be understood as a contextual and fluid *practice* (Cohen 2013, p. 1908). We may feel secure in discussing our health status with our doctor, but less so making disclosures to a market researcher who is surveying customers for a new over-the-counter remedy.

Helen Nissenbaum notes that with online data collection in the Age of Big Data, the context of informational consent is deeply flawed and increasingly meaningless (Nissenbaum 2011, p. 35). For many of us, most of our daily lives are enacted online, from filling out online job applications to creating bank transactions and communicating with loved ones. In a databased society, even if we do not interact digitally ourselves, maybe we choose to be off the grid, our information has a way of becoming digital regardless. Nissenbaum observes that we have little choice in this; we are increasingly forced to forfeit our informational privacy, and the transactional costs never favor us (2011, p. 36). If the liberal notion of privacy rights means that we should be able to control the context within which information about us is collected, used, and disseminated, this has always been a legal fiction in the USA. One only needs to consider this country's history of colonization and slavery, or the Federal Bureau of Investigation's COINTELPRO surveillance of the Black Panthers, The American Indian Movement (AIM), feminist organizations, and The Young Lords, among many other social justice groups, to understand that most Americans have never controlled the boundaries of their privacy (Flaherty 1989; Cunningham 2004). Certainly, this fiction is more poignant and insidious under the pall of digital technologies, Big Data, and the Patriot Act.

The notion that privacy entails the right to control either the conditions within which information on us is collected or how that data will be subsequently used, at least within healthcare settings, is an elusive one. We do not have the right to control the context of information collection, how it is stored, nor what is done with our data once we cede it to our doctor. In Chapter 4, I provide a deeper analysis of what rights we don't have, but here it is enough to say that under HIPAA's privacy regulations, patients must give authorization for third parties to use their data for marketing purposes and for disclosures not related to "healthcare operations." But this authorization is limited to the very narrow context of the doctor's office. A doctor or clinic cannot sell a patient's data for explicit marketing purposes without the prior, written consent of the patient. Yet, once patient data is moved out of the healthcare setting (under HIPAA this is called the "covered entity"), the patient's right to consent dissolves. This is what most often happens, as HIPAA's ultimate goal is to make data mobile.

In many other contexts, we have no rights over how our data is collected, stored, disclosed, or used in the larger network that health data can traverse. There are several court cases that are illustrative of this tension between patients who produce data within a healthcare setting, where they believe their privacy is protected, and those who lay claim to health data ownership outside of that protected context. Two recent cases in particular, one a US Supreme Court case, *Sorrell v. IMS Health Inc.* (2011) and the other case, *Arthur Steinberg et al. v. CVS Caremark Corporation et al.* (2012), dismissed by the US Eastern District Court (Pennsylvania), demonstrate that while patients may produce private data within healthcare settings—in both cases, prescription data—once these data are shorn of the patient's identity and mobilized outside of the clinic, they become the property of third-party innovators of that data (Boumil *et al.* 2012; Sweeney 2011; Pearson 2011). In both these cases, the courts found in favor of the third-party companies, and not for the patients that were suing for control over their data or for their privacy rights.

There exists a stratum of companies that work as data intermediaries between pharmacies, health insurers, and pharmaceutical and medical device manufacturers that most patients (and even many healthcare professionals) know little about. These companies are sometimes identified as prescription drug information intermediaries (PDIIs), such as IMS Health Inc., the defendant in the 2011 Supreme Court case, and they collect prescription data through license and purchasing agreements with pharmacies. They then resell or relicense that data to analytics companies, pharmaceutical manufacturers, marketers, and other data resellers (Ornstein 2014). I discuss these third-party data innovators in greater detail in the following chapters.

In the USA, in fact, as illustrated in the instance of selling prescription data, our rights to privacy are quite limited, and in some sectors or with some categories of information, in fact, we have no privacy rights at all. Privacy is contextual both to what can be kept private and under what conditions. Legal scholar Anita Allen explains that Congress has enacted a patchwork jumble of privacy and data protection laws since the 1970s, including more than eighteen federal laws, with additional legislation at the state level. Far from protecting our privacy, these laws, in fact, enable us more easily to alienate or waive our privacy rights (Allen 2011, p. 156). Many Americans believe that the right to privacy is enshrined in the Bill of Rights, protected by the Fourth Amendment outlawing undue search and seizure and the Fifth Amendment outlawing forced self-incrimination in court (Allen 2011, p. 157). While the Constitution does not explicitly state that we have a right to privacy, the Fourth and Fifth Amendments are used in defense of that presumed right. However, these rights to privacy are rights from unwarranted breaches by the government, not from the private sector, which is regulated by fragmentary laws concerned with protecting the privacy of consumers within certain, but not all, sectors. The right to privacy is not universal in the sense that it only extends to certain dealings with government and law enforcement. In the rest of life, such as with healthcare or banking information, privacy rights are regulated sector by sector. This approach contrasts with many other countries and regions, including the European Union (EU), which use omnibus privacy legislation. Within the omnibus context, people become "data subjects" that enjoy strictly protected privacy rights across all sectors, compared with the USA where a handful of Federal and state laws provide privacy standards for only twenty sectors of the economy (Dyson *et al.* 2014). The significant contrast between the EU's omnibus laws and the US' sector-specific laws is one of mobility: under EU law, personal data cannot cross national boundaries, while under US law most personal data is highly mobile and traverses globally. Despite this, many Americans believe that our privacy rights are universal, and thus we have a say in how our information is collected, stored, shared, and disclosed. This may come from a moral sense of privacy rather a legal one (Allen 2008). In fact, we have no omnibus legal right to privacy.

Confidentiality is essential to cultivating trust between a patient and her doctor, as well as all the other professionals in the clinical setting that are concerned with providing her healthcare. A trusting relationship is important because without assurances of confidentiality, a patient may not be honest with her doctor about her health. This lack of trust can have a deleterious impact on the patient's health. The two-thousand-year-old Hippocratic Oath, taken by doctors around the world, is intended to engender trust in the doctor-patient relationship through the promise of privacy. When the World Medical Association codified the Hippocratic Oath in the 1948 Declaration of Geneva, they made confidentiality its fifth principle. All subsequent oath modifications maintain confidentiality, as it is one way that doctors promise to "do no harm" to patients (World Medical Association 1948). US privacy regulations determine what is permissible and impermissible disclosure of patient information. These laws often stand in direct opposition to the ethical guidelines and principles of medical practitioners. A doctor's disclosure of patient information through HIPAA can often contradict this core value in medicine—confidentiality—where doctors pledge to keep their patients' health and medical information guarded. It is within this fragmented and contradictory relationship produced by the law and reflected in practice, that doctors and nurses handle patient privacy in their day-to-day work, which I detail in Chapters 4 and 5.

The significance of protecting trust and privacy in the medical relationship is exemplified in the case of Blanca Borrego, an undocumented immigrant who has lived in the USA for more than a dozen years. Borrego was arrested in her gynecologist's office for using a fake driver's license as proof of identity (Hennessy-Fiske 2015). When Borrego went to her gynecologist, a doctor that she trusted to provide her with appropriate care for an ovarian cyst regardless of her immigration status, imaginably, her trust extended throughout the healthcare setting to include the office staff that collected her data. Borrego entered a social context that comes with a higher legal and social expectation of privacy—much like a church or a psychiatrist's office. Except in cases where the abuse of a child, elderly, or disabled patient is suspected, where healthcare practitioners are legally required to report their suspicions to authorities, within any healthcare setting, the expectation of privacy is assumed once a patient walks through the door. Suspicions concerning a patient's immigration status are not grounds to violate a patient's confidentiality.[4] For Borrego and other patients like her, the expectation one has when entering the hospital is not one of privacy but rather betrayal. Borrego's case highlights how the law requires doctors to violate the core principles of their professional practice.

Along with ensuring confidentiality in the medical relationship, the principle of informed consent and a respect for the autonomy and bodily integrity of the patient is also fundamental to professional and ethical medical practice (O'Neill 2002). The twentieth-century global codification of medical informed consent emerged from public revelations of shockingly unethical medical practices, research, and experimentation conducted on patients in the name of science (Rothman 1991). While many medical professionals were concerned with some version of informed consent in earlier periods, it was during the mid-twentieth century that its import came into sharp and urgent focus. In the years following World War II, a series of international conventions, laws, and procedures took shape in response to the egregious medical practices, such as vivisection or inhumane experiments performed on prisoners, revealed during the Nuremberg Trials, the Tokyo Trials and the Khabarovsk War Crime Trial that prosecuted researchers working at Unit 731(Faden and Beauchamp 1986). The global medical community, along with legislators and political leaders in many countries, found the need to delineate and codify consent within medical settings.

Within medical ethics guidelines, in order for a patient to give consent to her doctor for treatment, a few conditions need to be met. The first condition is that the patient is fully informed, through language that she can comprehend, of each procedure. This includes the procedure details, its risks to her health or chances of success or survival, and its potential health benefits. The second condition is a lack of coercion. The patient must make her treatment decision free of non-compliance penalties. The patient submits to treatments of her own will. The final condition that must be met is that the patient explicitly gives permission to the healthcare provider to perform the procedures as described to her (Faden and Beauchamp 1986, p. 54).

Another condition that should be met before a patient can give her informed consent for a treatment pertains to privacy in terms of both her diagnosis and her treatment. Within another document, the Helsinki Declaration, under the World Medical Association, within Section B, point 21 of the text ("Basic principles for all medical research") is explicit concerning respecting patient privacy:

> The right of research subjects to safeguard their integrity must always be respected. Every precaution should be taken to respect the privacy of the subject, the confidentiality of the patient's information and to minimize the impact of the study on the subject's physical and mental integrity and on the personality of the subject. (World Medical Association 1964)

Although the Helsinki Declaration concerns medical research, these ethical guidelines inform clinical practice as well. Part of the concern of the Helsinki Declaration and the Belmont Report, guidelines on conducting ethically sound medical research prompted in part as a response to the Tuskegee Syphilis Study made public in 1972, is the recognition of and respect for patient autonomy. All of these ethical guidelines put together over most of the twentieth century, demonstrate that respect and recognition in medical practice comes in part by recognizing and respecting patient privacy, including protecting patients' informational privacy. So when a patient gives informed consent to allow her doctor and nurses to perform particular procedures on her, is she also giving informed consent to her healthcare providers to use and share her private information in ethically sound ways? Most often, she is not.

Notwithstanding the legislation and clinical practices in place that ostensibly protect patient privacy, patients in the USA do not give informed consent to how their information is used or shared, as I discuss at length in Chapter 4. Patients are required to acknowledge that the practice's privacy regulations were presented to them, but they are not consenting to anything that the practice might do with their private data.

Biologically derived data, information that is fundamentally about who we are, is often considered a "form of intangible property," at least by patients and even healthcare providers, who co-produce and disclose this data. Significantly, since these data are produced and stored digitally, many who argue for health data privacy argue for digital personhood—just as we "own" our bodies, so too we "own" our data personhood. One such person is Hugo Campos, an "e-patient" advocate who wants patients to have access to the data their bodies produce through implanted medical devices such as pace makers. He points out, "[i]t's my body, my life, my health. Why shouldn't I have access to do as I please with this data?" (Standen 2012). As I discuss in Chapter 5 more extensively, US law does not recognize patients who produce health data as owning it, nor does the law provide them the right to access or profit from it, as the case of *Sorrell v. IMS Health Inc.* made clear. The power over health data and digital personhood has never been in the hands of the patient.

Notes

1. While abortion stories were certainly published in the pre-Internet days, for instance in *Our Bodies, Our Selves* (Boston Women's Health Book Collective 2011), there are now several online outlets in which women are disclosing their narratives of terminating a pregnancy. Some of these outlets include 1in3campaign.org, a page maintained by the National Abortion Rights Action League (www.prochoiceamerica.org/womens-voices/womens-stories/), and the Twitter hashtag #ShoutYourAbortion.
2. As both Kapsalis (1997) and Holloway (2011) argue, the control of women's reproduction has long been a matter of public interest in the USA. Kapsalis describes the invention of the modern speculum, perfected on non-consenting, enslaved Black women's bodies by Dr. J. Marion Sims (dubbed the "architect of the vagina"), and displayed on White women's bodies in public demonstrations. Holloway similarly describes the public control of women's fertility and reproductive capacities, especially within the economic context of slavery.
3. The *Los Angeles Times* reported in January 2014 that Seay, a bereaved father who had recently lost his teenaged daughter in a car accident, received marketing material from the office supply retailer OfficeMax addressed to "Mike Seay, Daughter Killed in Car Crash" as mentioned in Chapter 1 (Pearce 2014).
4. In a *Los Angeles Times* article about Borrego's case, a spokesman for the hospital system where Borrego's arrest occurred stated that while it goes against hospital policy to deny care to patients based on their immigration status, authorities were contacted because Borrego used a fraudulent ID card (Hennessy-Fiske 2015).

References

Acquisti, Alessandro, Laura Brandimarte, and George Loewenstein. 2015. "Privacy and Human Behavior in the Age of Information." *Science* 347 (6221): 509–14.

Ali, Joe, Celeste Lee, Donna Cryer, Bradley Malin, Deven McGraw, and Lisa Schlager. 2015. "Promoting Research While Respecting Privacy: The Promise and Challenge of Using Patient Healthcare Data in Research." Conference

Roundtable presented at the Health Privacy Summit, Georgetown Law Center, Georgetown University, Washington, DC, June 3. https://patientprivacyrights.org/2015-health-privacy-summit-agenda.

Allen, Anita L. 2008. "The Virtuous Spy: Privacy as an Ethical Limit." Public Law and Legal Theory Research Paper Series Research Paper #07-34. Philadelphia: University of Pennsylvania.

———. 2011. *Unpopular Privacy: What Must We Hide?* Oxford: Oxford University Press.

Arthur Steinberg, et al. v. CVS Caremark Corporation, et al. 2012, 899 F.Supp.2d 331. 2012. Pennsylvania: United States District Court, Eastern District.

Bahadur, Nina. 2015. "Why Women Are Shouting Out Their Abortion Stories on Twitter." *Huffington Post*, September 21. Accessed January 9, 2016. http://www.huffingtonpost.com/entry/women-are-tweeting-shoutyourabortion-to-end-abortion-stigma_55fffcf0e4b00310edf7a02c.

Balasanov, Yuri. 2015. "From Gauss to Google: 200 Years of Evolution of Data Science and Marketing Analytics." Data Marketing Association (DMA) presented at the Town Hall: Analytics and CRM Community, Chicago, July 8. https://www.youtube.com/watch?v=Rpra2DUhHDU&feature=youtu.be.

Barocas, Solon, and Helen Nissenbaum. 2014. "Big Data's End Run Around Procedural Privacy Protections." *Communications of the ACM* 57 (11): 31–33.

Benhabib, Seyla. 2007. *Situating the Self: Gender, Community and Postmodernism in Contemporary Ethics.* Cambridge, UK: Polity.

Borzutzky, Daniel. 2015. *In the Murmurs of the Rotten Carcass Economy.* New York: Nightboat. http://bombmagazine.org/article/6941/data-harbor.

Boston Women's Health Book Collective. 2011. *Our Bodies, Our Selves.* 5th ed. New York: Simon & Schuster.

Boumil, Marcia M., Kaitlyn Dunn, Nancy Ryan, and Katrina Clearwater. 2012. "Prescription Data Mining, Medical Privacy and the First Amendment: The U.S. Supreme Court in Sorrell v. IMS Health Inc." *Annals of Health Law* 21 (2): 447–91.

boyd, danah. 2014. "What Is Privacy?" *Danah Boyd - Apophenia*, September 1. Accessed January 9, 2016. http://www.zephoria.org/thoughts/archives/2014/09/01/what-is-privacy.html.

Brunton, Finn, and Helen Nissenbaum. 2015. *Obfuscation: A User's Guide for Privacy and Protest.* Cambridge, MA: MIT Press.

Cohen, Julie E. 2013. "What Is Privacy For?" *Harvard Law Review* 126: 1904–33.

Cunningham, David. *There's Something Happening Here: The New Left, The Klan, and FBI Counterintelligence.* Berkeley and Los Angeles: University of California Press, 2004.

Duster, Troy. 2003. *Backdoor to Eugenics.* New York: Routledge.

Dyson, Andrew, Jim Halpert, Thomas Jansen, Diego Ramos, Richard van Schaik, Scott Thiel, Carol A. F. Umhoefer, and Patrick Van Eecke. 2014. *Data Protection Laws of the World Handbook.* 3rd ed. Leeds, UK: DLA Piper.

Faden, Ruth R., and Thomas L. Beauchamp. 1986. *A History and Theory of Informed Consent.* Oxford: Oxford University Press.

Flaherty, David. *Protecting Privacy in Surveillance Societies: The Federal Republic of Germany, Sweden, France, Canada, and the United States.* Chapel Hill, N.C.: The University of North Carolina Press, 1989.

Fuchs, Christian. 2014. *Social Media: A Critical Introduction.* London: Sage.

Hennessy-Fiske, Molly. 2015. "Advocates Protest Latina Immigrant's Arrest at Texas Doctor's Office." *Los Angeles Times*, September 15. Accessed January 9, 2016. http://www.latimes.com/nation/nationnow/la-na-houston-immigrant-clinic-arrest-20150914-story.html.

Holloway, Karla F. C. 2011. *Private Bodies, Public Texts: Race, Gender, and a Cultural Bioethics.* Durham, NC: Duke University Press.

Kapsalis, Terri. 1997. *Public Privates: Performing Gynecology from Both Ends of the Speculum.* Durham, NC: Duke University Press.

Magill-Cook, Lori. 2015a. "Write-Ups on Experian's Newborn Network Database," August 4.

———. 2015b. "The New Parent Market Is Growing (and Spending)," December 5.

Marwick, Alice E., and danah boyd. 2014. "Networked Privacy: How Teenagers Negotiate Context in Social Media." *New Media & Society* 16 (7): 1051–67.

Merchant, Carolyn. 2008. "Secrets of Nature: The Bacon Debates Revisited." *Journal of the History of Ideas* 69 (1): 147–62.

Nass, Sharyl J., Laura Levit, and Lawrence O. Gostin, eds. 2009. *Beyond the HIPAA Privacy Rule: Enhancing Privacy, Improving Health Through Research.* Washington, DC: Institute of Medicine, Nation Academies Press.

Nissenbaum, Helen. 2011. "A Contextual Approach to Privacy Online." *Dædalus* 140 (4): 32–48.

O'Neill, Onora. 2002. *Autonomy and Trust in Bioethics.* Cambridge: Cambridge University Press.

Ornstein, Charles. 2014. "Big Data + Big Pharma = Big Money." *ProPublica*, January 10. Accessed January 9, 2016. http://www.propublica.org/article/big-data-big-pharma-big-money.

Pearce, Matt. 2014. "Dad Gets OfficeMax Mail Addressed 'Daughter Killed in Car Crash.'" *Los Angeles Times*, January 19. Accessed January 9, 2016. http://articles.latimes.com/2014/jan/19/nation/la-na-nn-officemax-mail-20140119.

Pearson, Sophia. 2011. "CVS Accused in Suit of Selling Customer Data to Drugmakers." *Bloomberg Business*, March 9. http://www.bloomberg.com/news/articles/2011-03-09/cvs-accused-in-suit-of-using-customers-pharmacy-data-for-drug-companies.

Professional Services Close-Up. 2014. "PatientsLikeMe Survey Indicates People With Health Conditions Are Willing to Share Their Health Data." *Professional Services Close-Up*, January. Accessed January 9, 2016. http://www.library.drexel.edu/cgi-bin/r.cgi/login?url=http://search.proquest.com/docview/1491872926?accountid=10559.

Rothman, David. 1991. *Strangers at the Bedside: A History of How Law and Bioethics Transformed Medical Decision*. New York: Basic Books.
Sagoff, Mark. 2012. "Data Deluge and the Human Microbiome Project." *Issues in Science and Technology* 28 (4): 71–78.
Solove, Daniel J. 2006. "A Taxonomy of Privacy." *University of Pennsylvania Law Review* 154 (3): 477–564.
Sorrell et al. v. IMS Health Inc., et al., 564 U. S.10-799 2011. Supreme Court of the United States 2011.
Standen, Amy. 2012. "Patients Crusade for Access to Their Medical Device Data." *NPR*, May 28. Accessed January 10, 2016. http://www.npr.org/sections/health-shots/2012/05/28/153706099/patients-crusade-for-access-to-their-medical-device-data.
Sweeney, Latanya. 2011. "Patient Identifiability in Pharmaceutical Marketing Data." Data Privacy Lab Working Paper 1015. Cambridge, UK. http://dataprivacylab.org/projects/identifiability/pharma1.html
Turow, Joseph, Michael Hennessy, and Nora Draper. 2015. *The Trade-off Fallacy: How Marketers Are Misrepresenting American Consumers And Opening Them Up to Exploitation*. A Report from the Annenberg School for Communication University of Pennsylvania. Philadelphia: University of Pennsylvania.
Vertesi, Janet. 2014. "My Experiment Opting Out of Big Data Made Me Look Like a Criminal." *Times*, May 1. http://time.com/83200/privacy-internet-big-data-opt-out/.
Warren, Samuel D., and Louis D. Brandeis. 1890. "The Right to Privacy." *Harvard Law Review* 4 (5): 193–220.
World Medical Association. 1948. *The Declaration of Geneva. World Medical Association*. Accessed January 9, 2016. http://www.wma.net/en/30publications/10policies/g1.
———. 1964. *The Helsinki Declaration. World Medical Association*. Accessed January 9, 2016. http://www.wma.net/en/30publications/10policies/b3.

CHAPTER 4

Coercive Consent and Digital Health Information

Most of us who access healthcare in the USA expect to receive a pile of forms when we check in at the front desks of our doctors' offices. As patients, we often do not give a second thought to the type of contractual and transactional relationship with our doctors, nurses, with the entire healthcare industry that we are consenting to when we seek out healthcare. Do we enter into an equitable relationship or is it, by nature of the institution, always asymmetrical? We walk into the clinic and we know the drill; we are very familiar with the rituals in which we are required to participate. This humble detective is no different.

As I returned to the seating area of the clinic's waiting room, I peeked at the forms that the medical assistant behind the check-in desk handed me. On top of the pile, there were two pages of pink paper dedicated to a checklist, a long list of symptoms. In the last month, have you suffered from headaches or blurred vision, do you have a family history of diabetes or heart disease? Check yes or no. The third page was different. It outlined the clinic's policies and practices in regard to how it shares my health information with other "covered entities." It emphasized that the clinic takes efforts to protect my privacy. The sheet was printed in blue ink on white paper, the ink had bled a bit around each letter, and the type appeared to be about a nine-point font. The text was formatted in bullet points containing brief single-spaced paragraphs. The form heading, in bold Helvetica typeface, was titled: "HIPAA: Notice of Privacy Practices." Below the heading was a subheading: "This Notice Describes How Medical Information About You May Be Used and Disclosed and

M.F.E. Ebeling, *Healthcare and Big Data*,
DOI 10.1057/978-1-137-50221-6_4

How You Can Get Access To This Information. Please Read it Carefully. Changes On This Notice Will Not Be Honored." I took that sheet more seriously than the others. There were three columns that ran its length. The first paragraph explained that the clinic was concerned about protecting my privacy, as required by law, and that they would only disclose my "protected health information (PHI)" as permitted by applicable law. The first two columns fell under the heading "Uses and Disclosures of Your PHI," the last one under the label "Rights That You Have."

Any good detective knows that the devil is in the details, sister, and any gumshoe worth her weight in data bits reads, closely and carefully, line by line before signing any official or binding document. But I was confused as to what exactly I was signing. Was it a consent form? Was this a legally binding document of some kind? If I didn't sign it, could my doctor still see me? A simple form tells me I should sign the sheet in acknowledgement that I have read the clinic's Notice of Privacy Practices (NPP). I looked into both the sheets for an explanation, but there was none.

Despite my anxiety about getting the forms completed quickly so that I could see the doctor soon and hopefully find some explanation of my inability to get pregnant, I read the NPP. It astounded me. The very title of the form was in direct conflict with itself. Was this a notice of the steps that the clinic takes to protect my privacy or was it telling me how it would use and *disclose* my private health information? The opening paragraph didn't clarify this confusion but only deepened it. The notice informed me that the clinic reserves the right to change the terms of the notice at any time. Before detailing how and when the clinic is legally permitted to disclose my PHI, the sheet informed me that, in particular circumstances, the clinic would not disclose or share my PHI unless I signed an authorization form. But the form accompanying the Notice of Privacy Practices said that by signing it, I *acknowledged* that I was given the clinic's NPP. It did not say anything about me giving authorization to the clinic to share my PHI. I didn't have the time to dwell on this in the waiting room, so I moved on to the uses and disclosures of my PHI. The sheet detailed three instances in which the clinic must obtain prior authorization before they disclosed my PHI: the release of psychotherapy notes, use of my PHI for marketing purposes by third parties, and the sale of my PHI. Furthermore, I was informed that my PHI would be shared with "covered entities" or third parties that are involved with the provision of my healthcare, although the form did not define who is a "covered entity," I assumed it was another part of the hospital system or maybe my health insurer, but I wasn't sure.

I was also informed that my PHI could be shared with certain entities that were not "covered" for certain purposes, such as when the clinic contracts with third-party businesses.

The paragraph titled "Other Uses and Disclosures" piqued my attention. It read: "We are permitted or required by law to make certain other uses and disclosures of your PHI without your consent or authorization. Subject to conditions specified by law: We may release your PHI for any purpose required by law." Was this an informed consent form protecting my private data or a form acknowledging that the clinic allowed me to read their NPP? Exactly what was I consenting to? Another paragraph deepened my anxiety:

> Restrictions on Use and Disclosure of Your PHI. You have the right to request restrictions on certain of our uses and disclosures of your PHI for treatment, payment or healthcare operations. A restriction request form can be obtained from the doctor's office or hospital that you visited. *We are not required to agree to your restriction request, unless otherwise described in this notice, but we will attempt to accommodate reasonable requests when appropriate and retain the right to terminate an agreed-to restriction if we believe such termination is appropriate.* In the event that we have terminated an agreed upon restriction, we will notify you of such termination. (my emphasis)

Dejected by the realization that, in essence, I had no rights to control my data, I returned to the front desk administrator in a last-ditch effort to ask for help in understanding all of this paperwork. She had stepped away from the desk, so, not knowing what else to do, and mindful that I needed my doctor's and the clinic's assistance to make a much-wanted baby, I left my pile of paperwork, completed and reluctantly signed, on the desk.

My doctor's privacy notice, I found out later, is fairly typical in its incomprehensibility. In their analysis of Notices of Privacy Policies from the top 185 hospitals in the USA, for instance, public health researchers Peter Breese and William Burman determined that 183 of the 185 NPPs studied scored fairly to very difficult to read, using the Flesch Reading Ease Formula, with 92 percent of the notices requiring a patient to be in possession a PhD-level education to understand them (Breese and Burman 2005, p. 1593). Notwithstanding the fact that I do have a PhD, I found that not only could I *not* understand my doctor's notice, I discerned a malevolent intent behind its ambiguous and obfuscating language—its real message was a threat of disclosure. The true meaning of the notice's message is that I have no rights or control over my health data, that the data produced by my health status, by my own body, in collaboration with doctors, nurses, and medical billing professionals, are not mine. By virtue of that fact, I have little to no say in how, when, or to whom my data will be disclosed. While the document's title implies that the text will discuss privacy, not once in the text is it said that any of my data will be kept private—just the opposite. The document lists all of the ways and with whom my data may be *shared*. The notice uses "doublespeak" language that "pretends to communicate, but really does not," shifting responsibility away from the institution and onto the patient, and reinforcing the asymmetry of the relationship (Lutz 1989, p. 4). Through the text's doublespeak, the document embodies all of the heft and power of the medical institution, backed and endorsed by the law.

If the function of such a text, these documents produced within bureaucratic systems, is to connect local social relationships to larger structural forces, then this NPP is the embodiment of the clinic's objective institutional power over my data. Sociologist Dorothy Smith (2001, 2005) describes the power that texts have in reinforcing the sociopolitical interests of the greater system (including financial interests), all the way down to how people are to relate to one another in a doctor's office. She describes texts as "key devices in hooking people's activities in particular local settings and at particular times into the transcending organization of ruling relations" (Smith 2001, p. 164). The NPP emphasizes that the ways in which the clinic possibly will use and disclose my private health data are all permissible *by law*, thus linking local medical practices to the larger legislative bodies that have already determined how I am to relate to my doctor. But implicit in the text as well is how the practice of disclosure is fundamental to the healthcare industry's commercial and political interests. In fact, I argue that the NPP is the embodiment of the commercial interests of the American healthcare system.

Despite the document's doublespeak, in fact *because* of it, the ruling relations behind the clinical interaction are made clear: By agreeing to receive medical support through the clinic, I am also ceding control over any data that is produced out of that relationship to the clinic (Smith 2005, p. 119). While I may have some rights, at least as it is stated in the column labeled "Rights You Have," to control portions of my health record or to whom some of my data might be disclosed, the clinic reserves the ultimate right to ignore my requests for control. The menace embodied in the NPP raises questions about what kind of informational or "data" relationship

I have with my doctor and the entire healthcare system since I know that my data will be shared—at a minimum—with my health plan and with the pharmacy that will fill my prescriptions. How does the data image created from my health record differ from who I actually am as patient, as a human being? Will the healthcare system, and those who are charged with my care, interact with my data image first rather than with me? How will my health data image be used in other contexts, such as in combination with my Fair Isaac Corporation (FICO) credit risk score or other matrices, such as Experian's Mosaic marketing segmentation described in Chapter 2? These instruments are no longer used to merely assess the potential financial risk of a client; credit and consumer scores are now used to render citizens legible in the databased society. Without a FICO score one is invisible. And how much more powerful such scores will be enriched with a person's health data.

The purposeful ambiguity of the NPP, with its implication of perilous doom, leaves me doubting what I am consenting to, and moreover, makes me seriously question if I even have the power to consent. While medical consent can be ambiguous and problematic (is it ever possible for a patient to truly understand all potential risks?), nonetheless there is a consent process involved that includes informing the patient and seeking permission from her before a cut is made or a needle punctures her flesh (O'Neill 2003; Rose et al. 2005; Konow 2014). Yet with the case of health data gleaned from my body, before I even sit down face-to-face with my doctor to share with her information about my health, before I allow her to touch my body, take tissue samples, or collect biometric data such as the weight of my flesh, the rate of my pulse, or my blood pressure, the NPP presents me with an asymmetrical power relationship. This relationship is overdetermined by the financial and political interests of the healthcare system (Rothman 1991). I am not informed of all of the dangers and risks that disclosing my data may entail nor am I asked for my permission to disclose my information by the clinic. I do not have the opportunity to consent.

Patient Privacy and the Elimination of Informational Consent

What are the institutional "ruling relations" that brought the NPP into being? How are patients and health professionals to navigate this text? To answer these questions, we need to understand how institutions define, through legislation and through social practice, terms like "privacy," "consent," "trust," and "security." These definitions are currently governed by the Health Insurance Portability and Accountability Act (HIPAA), as well as the several amendments to HIPAA and subsequent laws, including the Privacy, Security and Omnibus Rules. NPPs carry all the institutional baggage that cascade down from this legislation. As I argue in this chapter, HIPAA legislation and the health privacy laws that followed were not designed to protect patient privacy. Rather, they were designed to create a regulatory information system that can securely *disclose* patient data for the necessary functioning of healthcare provision and medical capitalism. HIPAA legislation created a secure system through which health practitioners could get paid for providing medical services, fraud could be caught, and payers—health insurers as well as Medicare and Medicaid—could control the healthcare provisioning through the use of health informatics to determine what patients should be allowed what procedures and at what cost. HIPAA is a deeply contradictory piece of legislation, at least in the eyes of health practitioners who handle patient data every day. These practitioners have direct contact and intimate medical relationships with patients, and therefore, are often the most diligent protectors of patient privacy. Because of this, however, they are also the most vulnerable to penalty when structural contradictions produce data breaches or disclosures that harm patients.

Congress passed the HIPAA in August 1996. Initially, HIPAA established guidelines for three areas: (1) the portability and continuation of health insurance plans for workers who lose or change their jobs; (2) medical insurance fraud and waste; and (3) the standardization of administrative procedures, especially regarding electronic health records and billing (Ali Pabrai 2003, p. 4). At the time that HIPAA was drafted, the expansion of electronic health records was growing exponentially and health professionals and regulators became concerned about developing privacy standards for the collection and transmission of digital records (Nass *et al.* 2009, p. 63). These concerns over patient data privacy were not reflected in the passed legislation, however. HIPAA's 1996 version contained no provisions in its 168 pages[1] guaranteeing the privacy of patient health data or providing informed consent to patients as to how their data could be used and disclosed. While the legislation provided *recommendations* for standards regarding patient privacy, as well as a mandate to clarify what data privacy rights patients should be entitled to (in Section 264, subsections A through C), the statute did not delineate patient privacy rights nor did it require providers to obtain consent to disclose information (104th

Congress 1996: vol. 1936, pp. 2033–34).[2] It took legislators close to two decades, until 2013, to refine and delineate the data privacy and security regulations. In 1996, the statute emphasized data security over patient informational privacy, especially the security of digital records in the context of fraud detection and reporting. This awareness of informational security's importance was evident particularly in the sections about the standardization of administrative procedures (such as billing), because those processes inherently involved private patient data and, increasingly, those data were digitized. For HIPAA's drafters, digital information posed more data security risks than paper records. Sociologist Amitai Etzioni observes that at the time that HIPAA was passed, the drive toward electronic health records and the creation of networked databases, along with the collection and dissemination of health data digitally, increased health data surveillance for reasons other than individual or public health benefits. Etzioni notes that by the early 1990s, health insurers were already collecting non-clinical patient data to deny coverage, and third-party companies like credit bureaus and data marketing firms were linking lifestyle data collected online to individual patients (Etzioni 1999, pp. 142–43). The new ability to link and mine an individual's health data across several sectors, unlike in the previous era of paper-based record keeping, was already a great concern among privacy scholars and patient advocates. Yet privacy, as far as legal scholars define it, is concerned with an individual's *right to control* how personal information is collected, used, and disclosed, and under what conditions this happens (Allen 2011). Because HIPAA focused on securing data to *enable* its disclosure, to prevent insurance and other types of fraud above all else, the law did not provision patients with a right to control whether or how their private health information was collected, used, or disclosed, nor did it provide patients the right to determine the conditions of how these processes occurred. As described in Chapter 3, a patient's ability to control the conditions of these three activities are essential to meeting the minimum standards of informational privacy.

The bill's "administrative simplification" provisions[3] instructed the US Department of Health and Human Services (HHS) Secretary to regulate how electronic patient health data should be transmitted, disclosed, handled, and stored. The simplification process added another layer to HIPAA's implementation, as its Privacy Rule is administered through the HHS Office of Civil Rights. The fact that the Privacy Rule is adjudicated through the Office of Civil Rights, rather than some other administrative unit, is telling; the Privacy Rule is understood legislatively as a basic patient right. The Privacy Rule regulations created a special class of data that is to be handled with particular care: the PHI, the identifying information connected to each patient and her health.

Protected health information includes eighteen points of data, including a patient's name, date of birth, gender, age, diagnoses, procedural codes,[4] and zip code, among other information that can be used to identify an individual. In November 1999, the HHS published the Privacy Rule draft with an informational consent clause, and opened the proposed legislation to public comment until February 2000. Within that commentary period, the HHS received more than 52,000 comments from the public. These comments informed the final Privacy Rule, published in December 2000, which required patient consent for health practices to disclose the patient's PHI (US Department of Health and Human Services 2003b, p. 4). However, as laws are living things, the Privacy Rule didn't last in this format for long and underwent more revisions and additional public commentary periods until the bill was finalized in August 2002, with a compliance deadline for most health systems and plans by April 2003. Thus, for relatively brief period under HIPAA, patients were able to give consent to how their PHI could be used and disclosed by their doctors, health plans, and other entities involved with their healthcare provision. The finalized 2002 Privacy Rule *eliminated* the informational consent requirement (Sobel 2007, p. 41). For a period of a little less than three years, patients enjoyed the right to say whether or not they agreed to how and under what conditions their private health data would be used and disclosed. While some health practices do give patients informational consent forms that claim that if the patient refuses to sign the form, the practice will not be able to treat the patient, this is in direct contradiction with regulations.[5] This is just a further indication that practices are not only confused about what the regulations require in regard to informational consent but also that some healthcare practitioners use similar tactics to obtain consent that companies such as Google, or Facebook or Experian use to obtain data from users.

When you sign a HIPAA authorization, which you are actually not legally required to do, you are agreeing that you were given a copy of the NPP and that your signature is an *acknowledgement* that the clinic gave you a copy. You are not authorizing anything with the signature. Furthermore, a patient cannot be denied healthcare services if she refuses to sign any HIPAA or NPP form given to her by her doctor.

Informed consent is what strengthens trust in medicine, especially in light of medicine's historical (and contemporary) horrific violations of patient trust, as I outlined in Chapter 3. For most health practitioners, informed consent is a process, a conversation that goes beyond a signature on a document. Bill Knowles, an orthopedic surgeon who has worked in a community hospital for twenty years, argues that informational consent should be treated like this, but he notes that there is no informed consent procedure for a patient to understand what will happen to her data, much less for her to agree to it:

> There is no such requirement for anybody to explain the content of a HIPAA authorization to the patient. Not the secretary at the front desk, not the doctor. ...'Can you explain to me what this says on page four?' Even the orthopedic surgeon might not understand it. ... [T]here is no informed consent process for HIPAA. ... [F]or clinical care, if you're coming in for, again I'll say a knee replacement, everything will be about the knee surgery. There's nothing in the informed consent for the surgery that has to do with oh, by the way, how will your data be used if it's shared. That's an entirely business relationship that is done through the HIPAA authorization.

These conditions and the ruling relations embedded in the NPP create a coercive environment for protected health information to be disclosed.

Networks of Disclosure Under the Three Rules

Through the final Privacy Rule, the HHS created several classes of regulated and legally accountable subjects. The first is the "consumer," which is the term the HHS used for "patient." This moniker signaled how legislators, health practitioners, and patients themselves were (and continue) to understand the market relationships that define the American healthcare system (Ebeling 2011; Cohen 2003). The second is the "covered entity," organizations such as hospitals, doctors' offices, healthcare clearinghouses, and health insurers, that either produce, handle, disclose, or disseminate PHI in electronic form. Thus, HIPAA combined and "covered" these varied entities under its privacy regulations. Through the creation of covered entities, regulators attempted to streamline the informational *disclosure* process, so that once a patient's health data was produced within a covered entity as an electronic health record (EHR) it could then more easily be shared or disclosed to other covered entities. Ostensibly, because a patient's record was created under the HIPAA umbrella, the data was presumed to be "protected" and the patient's PHI would remain private as long as it remained within the network of covered entities. Through HIPAA's covered entities data system, data privacy rights shift from the body of the patient upward to the covered entities—the healthcare providers, the health insurers, and others who handle the patient's PHI within the "closed system." This shift is very apparent in the move from paper to digital records as it entails a reconceptualization of privacy and security of the entire digital system, not just the privacy of a single paper record.

The third class of accountable subjects created by HIPAA are "business associates" that are not covered entities, per se, but are involved nonetheless in providing ancillary healthcare services, such a prescription benefits management company or legal counsel for a health insurer. The law assumes that business associates come into contact with patient electronic health data through disclosures made by covered entities (US Department of Health and Human Services 2003a). The services that these third-party businesses provide, such as medical transcription, often are essential to healthcare provision by the covered entity, but it is considered more efficient—and cheaper—for covered entities to outsource these services rather than do them in-house. As is the case with manufacturing, software, and other information technologies industries, increasingly these services are conducted overseas at a fraction of the costs of doing the work in-house or even within the USA.

To give a sense of the complexity and opacity of the network that digitized patient data traverses, let us consider the network's size. The HHS estimates there are more than one million healthcare providers and two million health plans that span the USA, all of which are considered "covered entities" (Office of Civil Rights (OCR), HHS 2003, p. 8364; 2013, p. 5567).[6] To understand the breadth and depth of the third-party, ancillary businesses that comprise the supply chain within the American healthcare industry, much less the entire network that electronic patient data potentially moves through, is a much bigger challenge. The HHS estimates that the number of business associates that possibly handle a patient's PHI is upwards of 500,000 (2013, p. 5567).[7] Through the contractual arrangements made between covered entities and their business associates (e.g., the contracts between a hospital and its legal counsel), the latter are bound to the same regulatory standards as the covered entity with regard to handling a patient's PHI. In other words, a business associate that handles a patient's PHI faces the same penalties as a covered entity if data is breached or mishandled.

In the early 2000s, the healthcare network and its digital data became increasingly complex, due to changes in networked computing and the structures of healthcare provision, such as the proliferation of managed care (Conklin 2002; Plsek and Greenhalgh 2001). In response, regulators and legislators wanted to add an amendment to HIPAA to standardize digital health records. The Security Rule, passed in February 2003, was the answer. It regulates how digital health records can be disclosed, how they must be stored and protected both physically and technically, and stipulates the security standards for covered entities that are responsible for producing, disclosing, storing, and sharing protected health information electronically.

The Privacy Rule created new classes of regulated subjects; the Security Rule created new classes of regulated data objects. For the next several years, covered entities were regulated by both the Privacy Rule and the Security Rule, and these legal measures standardized how they produced, transmitted, stored, and secured electronic patient records. Through these rules, covered entities were legally accountable to the HHS Office of Civil Rights and, in the case of breaches, would be fined (depending on the severity of the leak, sometimes millions of dollars). Business associates, by law, are not covered entities, but nonetheless, were made accountable to covered entities through the contractual obligations with which they provided services. If there was a breach of privacy concerning electronic patient records along the supply chain, prior to new laws passed in 2013, the HHS would sue the covered entity, not the business associates. The contracts that the business associate entered into with covered entities stipulated that business associates must comply with the same privacy and security standards as the covered entities. This system lasted until 2013, when new rules were developed out of economic stimulus legislation.

In the wake of the largest global economic crisis since the Great Depression, the Obama Administration implemented the American Recovery and Reinvestment Act of 2009 (The Recovery Act) in an urgent, legislative effort to stimulate the economy and pull flagging localities out of recession. Through the Recovery Act, the Health Information Technology for Economic and Clinical Health (HITECH) Act also was passed, and at the time of the bill's passage it granted \$19.2 billion in resources to the healthcare system to implement requirements. The HITECH Act was widely described as a way to modernize the nation's health information infrastructure, in which many healthcare providers still kept paper medical records. In many ways, the Act embodies technological optimism—technologies can solve national economic challenges—yet the law also represents the entanglements of corporate interests in legislation.[8]

The HITECH Act mandated the creation of a nation-wide electronic health data infrastructure to enable the unhindered flow of medical records.[9] It also required all healthcare providers to convert paper records into electronic ones, threatening stiff penalties to those providers that do not demonstrate "meaningful use" of electronic health records by certain dates. In doing so, this Act became a windfall for the electronic records industry, as well as helped to create new companies and products aimed at helping providers become HITECH- and HIPAA-compliant. The HITECH Act also compelled all medical practices, from independent physicians' practices to community hospitals with less than 300 beds to large, for-profit hospital systems, to completely transition to digital health records by 2015. For practices to be compliant, this required enormous capital investment, upwards of $19 million for a small hospital, and a loss of productivity, as employees had to shift their attention away from the day-to-day operations of a health practice toward entering paper record data into computerized systems (Menachemi and Collum 2011, pp. 51–52). In Chapter 5, I discuss in more detail how the HITECH Act empowers the EHR industry to own patient data.

The Omnibus Rule,[10] presented to the public by HHS in January 2013 as the final rule on privacy protection and data security standards under HIPAA, emerged from the HITECH Act. The Omnibus Rule was passed to tighten up certain patient privacy issues that the HHS claimed slipped through the legal gap between the Privacy Rule and the Security Rule (HHS Press Office 2013). Yet, considering that the Privacy Rule really is not about privacy in the first place, but about ensuring that patient data is "secured" for disclosure, perhaps we should consider the Omnibus Rule as the final say on the security of data, rather than on patient informational privacy. Since our purpose here is to understand the ruling relations of patient informational privacy as embodied in the NPP, I will focus on only those aspects of the final rule. The Omnibus Rule states that patients have a right to request a copy of their digital health record in electronic form, and that covered entities must obtain a patient's permission before they can sell a patient's PHI. It also tightened the rules on how a patient's PHI can be used for marketing or fundraising purposes. Despite these provisions, there are many more third-party entities, such as credit card companies and ARC® Inc., the fertility medical financing company mentioned in Chapter 1, that do not fall under the Omnibus Rule or HIPAA regulations.[11] These entities can still easily receive, disclose, buy, and sell protected health data. And this is exactly what happened with regard to my health information; my marketing baby was created through this loophole in this highly fragmented and confusing legislation, a loophole that isn't coincidental but built into the structure of the law itself.

Bill Knowles, the orthopedic surgeon that we met earlier in the chapter, notes how clinical patient data that is protected under HIPAA can be released without the patient's or the doctor's knowledge to third parties outside of HIPAA regulations:

> I can tell you from the clinician's point of view, the intent is to look at their data and examine their data so that they can improve the care they give their patients. Unless you belong to Kaiser Permanente, most small practice doctors don't have the computer networks and ... these big drug companies and these big medical device companies all do. ... [M]edical device companies are very sophisticated. While they want to make the right products for their subjects, they also want to do everything that Facebook does. They want to study this big data and use it for marketing purposes. They may say to the doctor and to the patient, we'll use the [data of] our business partners and you'll have no concept of who their business partners are. Even if it is within the one company, these companies are gigantic international corporations with all sorts of subsidiaries. They may use it for all sorts of stuff only peripherally related to the surgery that they've had. ... Just like Facebook is trying to take data that we give it voluntarily, and then figure out who they can sell the data to that it targets. That's my thoughts on how clinicians might be sharing the data [unknowingly with third parties].

Bear in mind that portions of these data that are collected by a data broker, such as an inferred diagnosis based on online search terms or a health provider visit, or a web user's name and other identifying information scraped by brokers, coincide with a patient's PHI and can be triangulated to pinpoint that individual (Libert 2015). During my conversation with data broker Doug Sheehan, who works for an aggregator that sells data to Wall Street's financial industry, he mentioned that while his firm was not "playing in the health data arena" just quite yet, they are trying to figure out how they can enter the field. For Doug's company, the way in is through medical devices:

> There's a number of different ways to try and get this information. One of the ways that we've looked at this in the past is working again with a company that serves, for example, the hospitals but using data other than the

> purpose of serving those hospitals. Maybe looking at an inventory software system in a hospital to understand their purchase habits. There's also other ways of doing it as well, satellite data looking at the number of trucks leaving a warehouse where you know medical device manufacturing facilities to be located.

While what Doug is describing is high-level data collection on the medical device industry through targeted analyses of specific manufacturers and hospitals, and not necessarily the clinical data collected by medical devices themselves, these aggregated data are sold and used for purposes other than the care of patients.

A portion of the Omnibus Rule is supposed to protect the PHI of patients that are self-paying, especially those patients who may have a health plan but choose to pay either cash or with some form of credit for certain healthcare operations. According to the final rule, patients may request that their healthcare provider does not disclose to their health insurer the procedures that they pay for out of pocket. For example, an HIV-positive patient may not want to have her status recorded in her health record, which will be shared with her employer-sponsored health plan. Even if a patient has health insurance or uses a single-payer plan like Medicare, some medical procedures or prescriptions are not covered by insurance and must be paid for by the patient. The data associated with these types of self-paying transactions are certainly collected by the doctor's office, pharmacy, the health insurer (if there is one), and bank or credit card company (if a card is used). Even if it is a cash payment, that transactional data is recorded by the doctor's office and possibly by the health insurer if the cash transaction is a co-pay. If a patient self-pays using her credit card, her monthly card statement will have the amount charged and the name of the doctor's office. The name of the clinic's specialty (e.g., cardiology) can also contain information about the procedure. All health services received at a doctor's office or hospital is data that becomes part of a patient's health record, both on the doctor's side and, more importantly, on the side of the bank or financial institution. Similarly, if a patient does online research about local clinics before making an appointment with a doctor, and this data is scraped by a data broker and sold to a marketer, these data and marketing companies also are not liable under HIPAA. Doug Sheehan, the data broker mentioned earlier, told me that one of the core datasets his company uses is the credit card transactional data of five million cardholders.

All of these businesses are not covered under HIPAA regulations, yet many of them regularly handle and trade in protected and identifiable health information. Moreover, while I discuss data ownership more thoroughly in the following chapter, it is important to note here that many credit card companies have agreements with data brokers to sell de-identified transactional data of millions of customers (including private health data) for data mining and predictive analytics purposes. These data sharing arrangements show how a patient's data becomes the "property" of the credit card company through the transaction, as well as how these data also become the property of the data broker.

An estimate of the total healthcare network's size cannot really account for all of the businesses that fall outside of HIPAA regulations and that potentially see parts of a patient's record or PHI. Health data privacy scholar Latanya Sweeney, developed a network map of covered entities, business associates, and third parties that may share or receive a patient's data. In her Data Map, Sweeney attempts to account for all of the possible nodes in which a patient's data record may pass through, including those entities outside of the HIPAA regulatory regime (see Fig. 4.1).

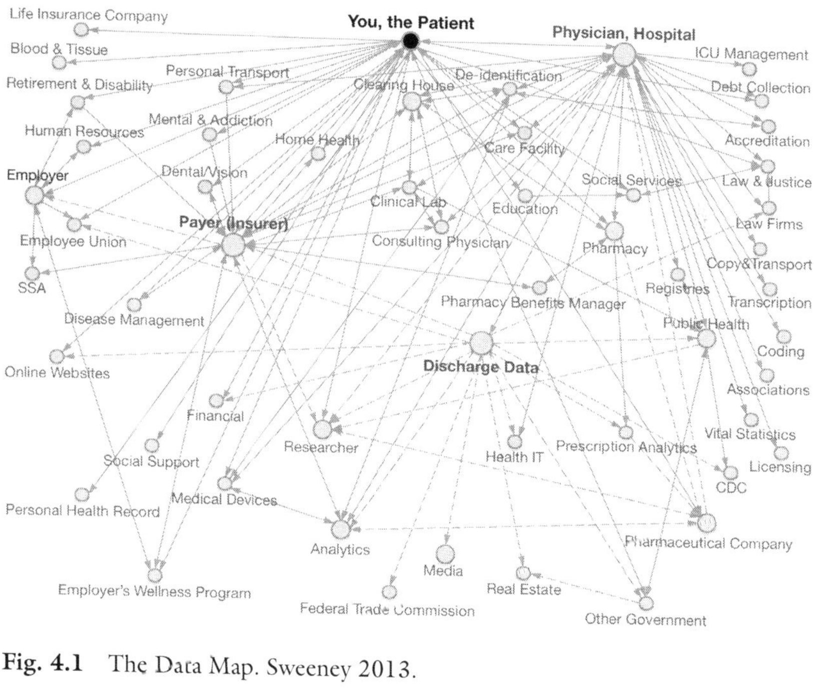

Fig. 4.1 The Data Map. Sweeney 2013.

Sweeney's Data Lab has also mapped how mobile phone software applications ("apps"), more than one hundred downloadable health and medicine apps, share a patient's PHI with third parties (Sweeney 2016).

In many ways, the total size and breadth of the network that comes into contact with a patient's private health data is too immense to quantify. When I asked the health professionals I interviewed if they knew how large the network is or how many people will handle patient data once it leaves their hands, most responded that they imagined "hundreds" of people may see a record, or at least parts of a record. No one could say for sure how many people may actually be able access an individual patient's private health information.

Privacy and Consent from Below

Empires are built through paperwork. Paperwork shapes material practices, even when there is not one scrap of paper to be found. In Ben Kafka's retelling of how the eighteenth-century neologism "bureaucracy" became the modern symbol of inscrutable and indifferent power, he describes how those who have do the paperwork, the "paper pushers" in government and industry, become the "thresholds of interpretation" of state and industrial power. Even if they remain critical interpreters, their work is to translate that power downwards through their paperwork (Kafka 2009). Similarly, in healthcare settings, doctors, nurses and healthcare administrators translate the power of the network of disclosure downward to the patient, even as they themselves are subjects of that power.

What does informational consent and privacy mean to the people that work with patients and their data day in and day out? For the majority of the health professionals that I spoke with, and especially nurses, privacy means HIPAA. In practice, the legislation represents regulations about data disclosure, and not necessarily about patient privacy (Sobel 2007, p. 40). During my interview with pediatric oncologist Tim Oberg, he argues that, in fact, it is a good thing that informed consent is not given for a patient's data or information, as it would be a breach of medical ethics to give informed consent for something as complex as how data is used and shared within medicine.

For many health workers who handle patient data on a daily basis, the acronym HIPAA is shorthand for the steps that they must take to protect patient privacy. I find this cultural practice very curious, considering that HIPAA was designed to enable the sharing and disclosing of patient health data, not about keeping patient data secret. In fact, the Notice of Privacy Practices that I describe at the beginning of this chapter listed all the ways that my doctor's office would disclose my private health data. It said nothing about how it would *not* disclose my data and keep my health information in confidence.

Healthcare practitioners—the doctors, nurses, medical assistants, and technicians charged with caring for patients—are, in general, deeply concerned with providing high-quality care in the best interests of their patients. Along with this concern comes an abiding attentiveness to respecting the dignity and autonomy of patients, and protecting their privacy. While privacy is of utmost concern for providers in theory, in practice it becomes a much more fungible concept. Not a single health professional that I spoke with, including surgeons, general practitioners, pediatric specialists, and nurses, had read their own practice's Notice of Privacy Practices. Many expressed having a sense that patients were given something to read when they checked in at the front desk, and some recalled seeing the NPP posted within the hospital. Many, though, were unsure what actually happened during the check-in process. They were equally unaware of whether or not patients were giving consent for how their data might be used or if they were instead simply informed that their data might be shared. Despite their lack of knowledge of their practices' privacy policies, most expressed deep concern about protecting their patient's privacy, at least while under their care.

HIPAA and its three amendments created a data infrastructure to disclose and share the private health information of patients. This data infrastructure was created "from above," primarily by legislators, policymakers, and legal experts, with little input from those who have to translate policy into clinical practices "on the ground"—the nurses, medical assistants, residents, lab technicians, orderlies, surgeons, and physicians of various specialties involved with patient care. Through this construction, two seemingly contradictory privacy contexts, and two coterminous social realities, were created: a digital network emphasizing disclosure (albeit highly regulated in regard to data security) and a clinical standard emphasizing privacy.

The security practices of these two privacy contexts overlap at times—a nurse knows not to write his passwords on a sticky note and stick it to a monitor, and he knows to always click off a record once he is done with it. One oncologist mentioned that although he carries his laptop everywhere he goes, he keeps no data on it, and only uses his laptop as a portal to access de-identified datasets for diagnostic research through the hospital's secured virtual private network (VPN). Yet for those who are occupied with the immediate care of patients, the digital network is asymmetrically tilted against clinical attentiveness. All the care that a surgeon may take to ensuring patient privacy, by not talking about her patients in an elevator or by locking her computer with extra passwords, is rendered essentially meaningless with every bit of data that she enters into an electronic record. That data is captured, moved through the various nodes in the network, and sold by third-party businesses. Many healthcare professionals are aware that despite all of their privacy work within the controlled space of the hospital or doctor's office, once that data is entered into the digital network, that control is lost. Amelia Cook is an emergency-room registered nurse, and in our interview about her privacy practices, she described her awareness of this loss of control:

> But I mean, it's out there. It's like sort of like cookies on your computer. 'Wait a minute how do they know, all of sudden I was looking for this and now all these ads are popping up.' … [W]e go to Home Depot and buy something and then all of a sudden someone has my credit card information. So, it's all the same thing, how secure is health data that's electronic? How secure is it? Nothing seems very secure any more. … [I]nformation is out there, whether it is in this cloud or its in the Midwest in these big CPUs, but its still there that somebody could get to. I sort of operate that it's all out there for the taking. … So I feel like, … do people really care? Because we care once it happens but are people asking for copies of their HIPAA that privacy thing? And [to be] perfectly honest, I don't know what that thing says. Do we as healthcare providers …should I know what it says if somebody asks me about their information?

The nurses, doctors, and surgeons that I interviewed about how they handle patient informational privacy (every interviewee called this "HIPAA"), sensed a Sword of Damocles hanging over their clinical and research practice. Their first priority is the effective and ethical treatment of their patients, but this treatment is overshadowed by their requirement to secure and disclose private patient health data.

Inside the hospital or clinic, health practitioners co-produce and handle patient data almost every minute of their shifts. Most of the data ends up being digitized, even if the original data entry was conducted on paper. In the words of one physician I interviewed, "it is a cultural phenomenon" in which several doctors, nurses, admissions staff, and medical technicians input data and update chart notes, often on different devices that are connected to one digital platform, at least within mid-sized to large healthcare settings such as an urban hospital. Through this cultural work around data, practitioners actively and systematically conduct the translational labor necessary to decipher legislative data privacy regulations into clinical practices.

Cook is an emergency-room nurse, and her job involves long hours of providing bedside care to her patients. For every patient that she sees, she must access their health record using the EHR software, EPIC. Virtually all the patient data produced and held in her hospital are stored on servers on the hospital's campus, and accessible through the networked system. Before walking into a patient's room, Cook opens the patient's record to learn a number of things: the reason they are in the hospital, if they have a history of hospital visits, what kinds of medications they may be on, any lab work they had done, and baseline data concerning their present health condition including blood pressure, heart rate, and other vitals. When she walks into the room, she needs these data to provide good care to her patient. And her patients often will expect that she has knowledge not only about their present state of health but also the history of their diagnoses, allergies, and other key information. Her knowledge of these things ensures they can trust her to provide good medical care as well as demonstrates that she is dealing with the patient in front of her, and not a data image.

Many clinical settings have rituals around privacy that are formalized through such things as required annual or semi-annual HIPAA trainings and re-certifications. Such trainings are usually conducted through proprietary online, self-directed training software that produces a certificate when the training is successfully completed to go into the employee's personnel file.[12] There are also more informal privacy rituals, such as writing "subjective, objective, assessment and plan" (SOAP) notes—a method of clinical documentation in which providers can use coded language to convey non-medical information, such as a patient with a "difficult" personality, to the next attending physician or nurse, without violating the patient's dignity or privacy. When the next caretaker opens the SOAP notes, she does interpretive work, inferring meaning while protecting privacy.

In emergency room (ER) settings, where there is a much greater chance that conversations about a patient might be overheard or someone might see that a patient has been admitted by looking at a dry-erase white board, for instance, some practitioners have devised practices to address privacy. For example, some ER practitioners only write patients' initials on the white boards or only speak about cases in the break room, away from family members waiting outside. Everyone knows not to look up a patient's record if there is no immediate, clinical need to do so, especially if the patient is not in their immediate care, because digital platforms keep a record of each time a record is accessed and by whom. The penalties for a breach, which include a fine up to $50,000 and the possibility of being fired, are well known and steep enough to quell any temptation to look up a patient's record when one shouldn't be (Stebner 2013). Even if there is information in a patient's record regarding active medications that they are taking, a nurse or physician will always ask a patient's permission to call their pharmacy to get accurate information. Some EHRs even build in this informal, informational consent regarding medications: when a doctor downloads a pharmacy's medications list for a patient, a pop-up window asks the user to say "I agree that I have consent," which the doctor must click before the file can be opened.

Often the work of translating legislative regulation into clinical practice appears to shore up patient privacy against a constant threat of harm and exposure. In one of the hospitals where several of the practitioners that I interviewed work, there are signs posted as a constant reminder of the threat to patients' privacy, which attributed that threat to the sloppy practices of the practitioners themselves. I observed one sign in an elevator reminding staff not to discuss patient cases in the elevator or other public locations. The sign also explained the appropriate reporting protocol if one happens to overhear such an incidental disclosure: The reporting person should obtain the names of the speakers and report them to the hospital's compliance officer so that the offenders may be properly educated.

For all of their vigilance, many health practitioners are aware that private patient data, when digitized, has a way of becoming accessible to those who are not concerned directly with patient care. Sondra Burns, an attending pediatrician at a children's hospital emergency room, noted how this privacy aporia shapes her data privacy practices:

> Facebook has been around the entire time of my adult life, pretty much I'm of the generation that I know that everything I do electronically is tracked by somebody. So I'm not going to do anything on a computer that I don't want anyone to know about because somebody is always going to find out … there is no such thing as privacy, is kind of my … it would be nice if there were probably but I conduct myself as a physician as if there were no such thing.

Through formal and informal practices, health practitioners maintain privacy, but they also know that it is as futile as the security rituals that we all perform at airports (take off your shoes, take off your belt, empty your pockets, walk through the machine) because they have little power to protect a patient's data privacy beyond their immediate role within clinical practice. They have no control once the patient's information moves from the hospital room to the various laboratories, third-party transcription companies, billing offices, health insurers, third-party health services management companies, pharmacies, and data brokers.

Coercive Consent in Capitalist Healthcare

Anthropologist of bureaucracy David Graeber notes in his article, "Dead Zones of the Imagination," that bureaucratic institutions, including health facilities, are violent by their very nature, as they are extensions of state power. He explains that the "violence I'm referring to here is not epistemic. It's quite concrete. All of these are institutions involved in the allocation of resources within a system of property rights regulated and guaranteed by governments in a system that ultimately rests on the threat of force. 'Force,' in turn, is just a euphemistic way to refer to violence" (2012, p. 112). Graeber goes on to explain that this threat of harm is embedded in the everyday material practices of bureaucracies. Despite their banality and boringness, if we fail to cooperate with bureaucrats by, say, using a false ID to receive healthcare, as was the case for Blanca Borrego in Chapter 3, the state (and industry—the two are intertwined in late capitalism) will use its monopoly on violence to enforce the rules.

Political and legal theorists, including Mitchell Dean, John C. Scott, and Dean Spade, point to the creation of institutions that embark on the mass collection and standardization of data from populations—information on everything from people's finances and financial behaviors, to their sexual practices and eating habits and on. Such collection and standardization of population data serves the intertwined projects of biopower, caretaking, and surveillance (Scott 1999; Spade 2011, pp. 140–41; Dean 2012). Bureaucrats such as the administrators and enforcers of HIPAA and HHS Office of Civil Rights workers have the legislative backing and heft of state power and violence, which creates a context of coercive consent in regard to private health data.

"Coercion is defined as intentionally compelling someone to a choice at the threat of imposing a penalty for non-compliance" (Konow 2014,

p. 50), and the data network created by HIPAA legislation is a network of coercion. HIPAA's most coercive aspect is the lack of informational consent, but while the coercion does not happen at the level of everyday interactions between, say, an intake specialist and a patient, where the specialist becomes frustrated when a patient refuses to sign a HIPAA acknowledgement form. No, the coercive relationship is embedded in the entire context of HIPAA, and it is not only the patients, but those "paper pushers"—health practitioners in this case—who live in fear of privacy breaches. After all, practitioners face huge fines, job loss, and even possible jail time. The heft of the organizational structure behind clinical practices renders the entire structure coercive, for patients and for health practitioners alike. It is death by a thousand paper cuts.

The parallel network of disclosure and, as I demonstrate in the following chapter, of data *ownership*, however, contains built-in legal loopholes for data to slip out in ways directly benefiting private interests, such as IMS Health Inc. which makes money off the private health data of patients. Again, these legal data disclosures are coercive. Employee "wellness programs" are perhaps the most striking example of coercive disclosures of patients' private health information that can benefit private interests. The Affordable Care Act of 2010 (ACA) mandates that employers must provide these programs to their employees (111th Congress 2010).[13] For employees to receive a "discount" on their employer-sponsored or subsidized health insurance, they must sign up for a wellness program, which is often provided by a third-party company that financially benefits from each client enrolled. The enrollment process usually requires the employee to complete a survey about behavioral health information, such as eating habits, whether they smoke or drink, stress levels, and how much exercise they get during the week, as well as information on prescriptions, mental health, and whether the employee is undergoing a divorce. Often these survey data will be combined with biometric information either gleaned from a physical mandated as a condition of enrollment or taken from the patient's health insurance record. The combined information can have serious implications for the employee, both financially and in terms of their health privacy. A patient's health insurance premiums may increase, for example, if they are found to be non-compliant by not changing their diet if they are obese, or by giving up on smoking cessation programs if they are smokers. Furthermore, giving employers access to employees' private health data through a third-party wellness program has profound implications for workplace surveillance and patient-employee privacy.

Deanna Fei details this power dynamic in her book *Girl in Glass*, in wh she describes how the CEO of the company her husband worked "outed" her premature baby's medical expenses during a company-wide meeting, and blamed Fei's family for the increase in the rates of the company's health plan (Singer 2013a, b, c; Lewis 2015; Fei 2015). In contrast to the health practitioners working in the clinical context of privacy, those who work within the network of disclosure (like data brokers, insurers and third-party businesses who take advantage of loopholes in HIPAA legislation) make money when data moves out of the clinic and into their hands. Health practitioners face jail time for similar movements of data. Yet for data brokers, such disclosures are legal—they are not breaches but legitimate leaks—since the network of disclosure is built to allow disclosures that are financially valuable to third parties. Just as with their patients, medical practitioners are on the shorter end of the privacy stick in the asymmetrical relationship between health data and the network of disclosure. In the following chapter, I consider the network of health information disclosure constructed by HIPAA legislation and how property rights over data are claimed more closely.

Notes

1. HIPAA's amendments were much lengthier than the original bill, making the original legislation seem thin and direct. With the Privacy Rule and Security Rule measuring 115 pages, the regulations on Meaningful Use of Electronic Health Records measuring 700 pages, and the Omnibus Rule measuring 500 pages, the legislation regulating the proper handling of patient records overwhelms many health practitioners.
2. HIPAA Section 264, Subsection b, addresses the recommended establishment of standards that address what patient informational privacy rights should be and the creation of guidelines for patients to exercise those rights: "(b) SUBJECTS FOR RECOMMENDATIONS—The recommendations under subsection (a) shall address at least the following: (1) The rights that an individual who is a subject of individually identifiable health information should have. (2) The procedures that should be established for the exercise of such rights."
3. Given HIPAA's lengthiness, and its bureaucratization of healthcare practices, it can hardly be considered administratively streamlined or simple. The term "administrative simplification" is another example of doublespeak.
4. All of these procedures are categorized as the ICD-10-CM (International Classification of Diseases, Tenth Revision, Clinical Modification), a classification system for diagnoses and conditions, as well as their associated

medical procedures within clinical settings. It was developed by the World Health Organization in 1994, and has become the standard for the entire US medical system. The patient's PHI and the ICD-10-CM codes used to describe what happens during a doctor's visit are considered "protected" information, so her doctor and her health insurer must protect all of that information. Revisions to the process through which doctors and hospitals are reimbursed by Medicaid and Medicare, a process that is the bellwether of the entire healthcare system, mean that insurers no longer pay a per-service fee for the overall health outcomes of a patient.

5. Interestingly, during the writing of this book, one evening, I had a health emergency one, which landed me in the emergency room of the same medical system where I had received fertility treatments for years. Apparently in the haze of the emergency room, a nurse had me sign a single sheet of paper labeled "General consent to use and disclose Protected Health Information." The form's text explained that the medical system was asking permission to use and disclose my health information, that the information is identifiable and that it can be traced back to me, and that by signing this form I am consenting to the clinic's uses and disclosures that they will make of my private health data. Furthermore, the form explained by signing that I am also acknowledging that I have received the Notice. The form's last line read: "If you refuse to sign this consent form, we will not be able to treat you." I was told that I signed this form only months later when I returned to the hospital for a follow-up appointment related to my health emergency. Only then was I informed that I had consented to the hospital using and disclosing my private health information.
6. These estimates are revised versions of those published in a 2000 HHS report. In the 2000 report, the department estimated the number of covered entities to be around 600,000. This was directly affected by changes in the regulations. The number was revised to 700,000 in 2013.
7. This estimate is derived from the text of the Omnibus Rule, Section A Part 3, Table 1: *Estimated Costs of the Final Rule*. There, HHS estimates the total number of covered entities at 700,000 in 2013, with about 500,000 agreements with business associates providing ancillary services to covered entities.
8. In his 2011 State of the Union Address, President Obama relied upon this familiar trope when he declared that America will "win the future" by out-innovating India and China. Obama stated that: "[t]he first step in winning the future is encouraging American innovation. None of us can predict with certainty what the next big industry will be or where the new jobs will come from. Thirty years ago, we couldn't know that something called the Internet would lead to an economic revolution. What we can do—what America does better than anyone else—is spark the creativity and imagination of our people. We're the nation that put cars in driveways and computers in offices;

the nation of Edison and the Wright brothers; of Google and Facebook. In America, innovation doesn't just change our lives. It is how we make our living" (Obama 2011). In many respects, "Big Data" as an innovation-based industry is also being pitched as a technology that will win the future for the US economy. Social historians of science and technology have long noted the rhetorical link made by American policy makers, legislators, economists, politicians, and commercial leaders between technological progress driving economic prosperity and American exceptionalism, See, for example, Noble's *America by Design* (1977) or Berman's more recent *Creating the Market University: How Academic Science Became an Economic Engine* (2012).

9. The HITECH Act set forth a framework for a national health information exchange (HIE) that would require all healthcare providers to provide interoperable health data that can move.
10. The HIPAA Omnibus Rule is so called because it is encompassing all of the legislation developed in the Privacy Rule and the Security Act. It is not an omnibus privacy law that covers all sectors; it only covers the HIPAA regulated health and medicine sectors.
11. While financial transactions made within a clinical setting may not necessarily fall under HIPAA regulations, they do fall under the financial privacy requirements of the Gramm-Leach-Bliley Act (1999) that regulates how financial institutions, as well as service providers, must secure transactional and non-public personal information (Federal Trade Commission 2002).
12. One such platform, HIPAAtraining.com, promises to make compliance "fast, easy, and painless." See http://www.hipaatraining.com.
13. In November 2012, Proposed Rules were implemented through the ACA that directly address workplace wellness programs that are connected to group health plans (US Department of Labor 2012).

References

104th Congress. 1996. *Health Insurance Portability and Accountability Act of 1996. 110 STAT.* Vol. 1936.

111th Congress. 2010. *Patient Protection and Affordable Care Act (ACA)*. 42 USC 18001.

Ali Pabrai, Uday O. 2003. *Getting Started with HIPAA*. Boston, MA: Primer Press.

Allen, Anita L. 2011. *Unpopular Privacy: What Must We Hide?* Oxford: Oxford University Press.

Berman, Elizabeth Popp. 2012. *Creating the Market University: How Academic Science Became an Economic Engine*. Princeton, NJ: Princeton University Press.

Breese, Peter, and William Burman. 2005. "Readability of Notice of Privacy Forms Used by Major Health Care Institutions." *Journal of the American Medical Association (JAMA)* 293 (13): 1593–94.

Cohen, Lizabeth. 2003. *A Consumer's Republic: The Politics of Mass Consumption in Postwar America*. New York: Vintage.

Conklin, Thomas P. 2002. "Health Care in the United States: An Evolving System." *Michigan Family Review* 7 (1): 5–17.

Dean, Mitchell. 2012. "The Signature of Power." *Journal of Political Power* 5 (1): 101–17.

Ebeling, Mary. 2011. "'Get with the Program!': Pharmaceutical Marketing, Symptom Checklists and Self-Diagnosis." *Sociology of Diagnosis* 73 (6): 825–32.

Etzioni, Amitai. 1999. *The Limits of Privacy*. New York: Basic Books.

Federal Trade Commission. 2002. "In Brief: The Financial Privacy Requirements of the Gramm-Leach-Bliley Act." Policy Brief BUS53. Washington, DC: Federal Trade Commission. https://www.ftc.gov/tips-advice/business-center/guidance/brief-financial-privacy-requirements-gramm-leach-bliley-act.

Fei, Deanna. 2015. *Girl in Glass: How My "Distressed Baby" Defied the Odds, Shamed a CEO, and Taught Me the Essence of Love, Heartbreak, and Miracles*. New York: Bloomsbury.

Graeber, David. 2012. "Dead Zones of the Imagination: On Violence, Bureaucracy, and Interpretive Labor." *HAU: Journal of Ethnographic Theory* 2 (2): 105–28.

HHS Press Office. 2013. "New Rule Protects Patient Privacy, Secures Health Information." *Department of Health and Human Services*, January 17. Accessed January 9, 2016. http://www.hhs.gov/news/press/2013res/01/20130117b.html.

Kafka, Ben. 2009. "Paperwork: The State of the Discipline." *Book History* 12: 340–53.

Konow, James. 2014. "Coercion and Consent." *Journal of Institutional and Theoretical Economics* 170 (1): 49–70.

Lewis, Al. 2015. "It's Official: Employee Wellness Is a 'Scam.'" *Huffington Post*, April 17. Accessed January 9, 2016. http://www.huffingtonpost.com/al-lewis/its-official-employee-wel_b_7046652.html.

Libert, Timothy. 2015. "Privacy Implications of Health Information Seeking on the Web." *Communications of the ACM* 58 (3): 68–77.

Lutz, William. 1989. "Notes Toward a Definition of Doublespeak." In *Beyond Nineteen Eighty-Four: Doublespeak in a Post-Orwellian Age*, edited by William Lutz, 1–11. Urbana, IL: National Council of Teachers of English.

Menachemi, Nir, and Taleah H Collum. 2011. "Benefits and Drawbacks of Electronic Health Record Systems." *Risk Management and Healthcare Policy* 4: 47–55.

Nass, Sharyl J., Laura Levit, and Lawrence O. Gostin, eds. 2009. *Beyond the HIPAA Privacy Rule: Enhancing Privacy, Improving Health Through Research*. Washington, DC: Institute of Medicine, Nation Academies Press.

Noble, David. 1977. *America by Design: Science, Technology, and the Rise of Corporate Capitalism*. Oxford: Oxford University Press.

Obama, Barack. 2011. "Remarks by the President in State of Union Address." State of the Union Address transcript. Washington, DC: White House. https://www.whitehouse.gov/the-press-office/2011/01/25/remarks-president-state-union-address.

Office of Civil Rights (OCR), Department of Health and Human Services. 2003. *Health Insurance Reform: Security Standards; Final Rule. HIPAA*. Vol. 45 CFR Parts 160, 162, and 164.

———. 2013. *Modifications to the HIPAA Privacy, Security, Enforcement, and Breach Notification Rules Under the Health Information Technology for Economic and Clinical Health Act and the Genetic Information Nondiscrimination Act; Other Modifications to the HIPAA Rules. 45 CFR*. Vol. Parts 160 and 164.

O'Neill, Onora. 2003. "Some Limits of Informed Consent." *Journal of Medical Ethics* 29 (1): 4–7.

Plsek, Paul E., and Trisha Greenhalgh. 2001. "The Challenge of Complexity in Health Care." *BMJ* 323 (7313): 625–28.

Rose, Diana S., Til H. Wykes, Jonathan P. Bindman, and Pete S. Fleischmann. 2005. "Information, Consent and Perceived Coercion: Patients' Perspectives on Electroconvulsive Therapy." *British Journal of Psychiatry* 186 (1): 54–59.

Rothman, David. 1991. *Strangers at the Bedside: A History of How Law and Bioethics Transformed Medical Decision*. New York: Basic Books.

Scott, James C. 1999. *Seeing Like a State: How Certain Schemes to Improve the Human Condition Have Failed*. New Haven, CT: Yale University Press.

Singer, Natasha. 2013a. "On Campus, a Faculty Uprising over Personal Data." *New York Times*, September 15. Accessed January 9, 2016. http://www.nytimes.com/2013/09/15/business/on-campus-a-faculty-uprising-over-personal-data.html.

———. 2013b. "Health Plan Penalty Ends at Penn State." *New York Times*, September 19. Accessed January 9, 2016. http://www.nytimes.com/2013/09/19/business/after-uproar-penn-state-suspends-penalty-fee-in-wellness-plan.html.

———. 2013c. "Rules Sought for Workplace Wellness Questionnaires." *New York Times*, September 25. Accessed January 9, 2016. http://www.nytimes.com/2013/09/25/business/rules-sought-for-workplace-wellness-questionnaires.html.

Smith, Dorothy E. 2001. "Texts and the Ontology of Organizations and Institutions." *Studies in Cultures, Organizations and Societies* 7 (2): 159–98.

———. 2005. *Institutional Ethnography. A Sociology for People*. Lanham, MD: AltaMira Press.

Sobel, Richard. 2007. "The HIPAA Paradox: The Privacy Rule That's Not." *Hastings Center Report* 37 (4): 40–50.

Spade, Dean. 2011. *Normal Life: Administrative Violence, Critical Trans Politics and the Limits of the Law*. Brooklyn, NY: South End Press.

Stebner, Beth. 2013. "Kim Kardashian Baby: Six People Fired for 'Improperly Accessing' Medical Records at L.A. Hospital Where Reality Star Gave Birth." *New York Daily News*, July 13. Accessed January 10, 2016. http://www.nydailynews.com/entertainment/gossip/hospital-workers-fired-accessing-kim-kardashians-medical-records-report-article-1.1398107.

Sweeney, Latanya. 2016. "Personal Health Data." Research. *The Data Map*. http://thedatamap.org/index.php.

US Department of Health and Human Services. 2003a. *Summary of the HIPAA Privacy Rule: Business Associates*. OCR Privacy Brief. Washington, DC: US Department of Health and Human Services, Office of Civil Rights.

———. 2003b. *Summary of the HIPAA Privacy Rule*. OCR Privacy Brief. Washington, DC: US Department of Health and Human Services, Office of Civil Rights.

US Department of Labor. 2012. *Incentives for Nondiscriminatory Wellness Programs in Group Health Plans. Federal Rules—ACA 2010*. Vol. FR Doc No: 2012–28361. http://webapps.dol.gov/FederalRegister/HtmlDisplay.aspx?DocId=26492&AgencyId=8&DocumentType=1.

CHAPTER 5

The Biopolitics of Lively Data

One late autumn day, in the late stages of research for this book, I received a mysterious and somewhat curious email. At first, I thought it was spam. But as I investigated it, the missive revealed the boiled-down biopolitical problematics of private health data in the hands of marketers and data brokers. An email was sent to my free, web-based account that I use for personal communications, and the message was automatically categorized as "finance" by the email system.

I found the origins of the email concerning and I determined to get to the bottom of it. Who was "personalhealth@webmdhealth.com"? Though I have, in the past, visited the public WebMD website to look up symptoms in an attempt to self-diagnose (even this hard-boiled detective is susceptible to the occasional bout of mild hypochondria), I didn't recall signing up for a "personal health record." In fact, I had no recollection whatsoever of entering any identifying information into the WebMD platform. I knew better than to do that. In all my visits, I had only clicked through the website's pages.

Going against my better judgment about what to do when receiving an unsolicited email, I clicked on the link labeled "Click here to get to your member site." When I did, I was redirected to my health insurer's website, Independence Blue Cross (IBX). Phew, it wasn't spam. But concern quickly overtook my relief. Has my health insurer handed over my data to WebMD? Well, yes, apparently. The email is the result of a new business relationship between WebMD and my employer-sponsored health insurer, IBX. IBX brokered a deal with the NASDAQ-traded health information

M.F.E. Ebeling, *Healthcare and Big Data*,
DOI 10.1057/978-1-137-50221-6_5

services company to create a web-based, consumer-facing platform that allows policyholders, such as myself, to access their personal health data and insurance claims.

Being the thorough detective that I am, I clicked through all of the privacy policies that WebMD provided in the email. Although the WebMD policy made it clear that I did not have a choice in whether I would allow yet another information services company to access, secure, store, disclose, and analyze my private health data, the text tried to reassure me that their company takes my privacy and the security of my data very seriously. Yet, I only learned of WebMD's possession of my data after the deal was done.

This email illustrates how the network of disclosure created by Health Insurance Portability and Accountability Act (HIPAA) legislation (discussed in Chapter 4) stretches and distorts privacy and security to include third parties. What I demonstrate in this chapter is not how our patient privacy is at risk from security breaches, but rather how it is at risk from the normal, "business-as-usual" selling of patients' private data. I show the harm and pain that this network of disclosure can cause. Robert Gordon, a health information technologies expert, during an interview with me stated that "the system persists because the harm and pain that it causes is anonymous and dispersed." In this chapter, I give that suffering a voice.

Neither patients nor healthcare providers concerned about patient privacy have much power to control what happens to patient data. This is primarily because even though that data may be *about* us, we do not *own* it. And since we don't own it, we have little say in what happens to it. My concern here is a feminist one: Struggles over health data property rights have parallels in struggles over the ownership and commodification of bodies. Anne Phillips observes that while there is virtually global juridical consensus that human bodies are not property nor should body parts be sold or made into commodities, there are nonetheless thriving markets for both, from commercial surrogacy to the markets in oocytes and sperm (Phillips 2013, p. 2; Almeling 2011; Waldby and Mitchell 2006; Scheper-Hughes 2001). Following the work of feminist scholars such as Carole Pateman, Nancy Scheper-Hughes and Margaret Radin, Phillips underlines the slippage toward self-alienation when we think of our bodies as our property that we can rent or sell as we please in the marketplace. Instead, she suggests, we should be thinking of our bodily integrity and bodily labor capacities (what Catherine Waldby and Melinda Cooper call "biolabor"), such as the bodily labor a woman performs to donate her eggs to an infertile couple (Waldby and Cooper 2010; Pateman 2002;

Scheper-Hughes 2001; Radin 1996). Much of this biolabor, of course, is under- or un-compensated, financially or otherwise. Catherine Waldby and Melinda Cooper stress how women are particularly dispossessed of the surplus value that their bodies produce for the fertility medical industry, for example, the profit realized out of oocyte production (Waldby and Cooper 2010). For some feminist scholars, while we may not own our bodies or our tissues (and many US laws legislate declare that we do not "own" our bodies), we nonetheless "own" our biolaboring capacities (Phillips 2013). Can our biolaboring capacities extend to the data that our bodies produce?

In this chapter, I describe the property relationships between protected health data and the healthcare information industry, primarily third-party companies that have positioned themselves on the outer nodes of the HIPAA network of disclosure, such as electronic medical records software companies and health informatics enterprises. Here I hope to disentangle, or at least trouble, the complex web of the health-data biopolitical economy. I analyze how ownership claims are made through possessing data and transformatively innovating it, a process which yields new data assets. These assets are mobilized back out into the network of disclosure. This data ownership mandates a patient's dispossession of their biolabor—and any ownership claims they may try to make over their health data—to produce data commodities. I demonstrate how, for data brokers and aggregators of health data, data is only useful if it is mobilized as new assets.

To do this analysis, I utilize a biopolitical framework. Biopolitics here names a regime, a way of organizing social life and "nature" through capitalist socialization, in which "life itself becomes an object of technological intervention, and nature 'has become capital'" (Lemke 2011, p. 69). Life—tissues, cells, DNA, blood, and organs—and data that is produced by life become subject to and the object of capital's speculative power. Life is sliced up, mixed together, mined, instrumentalized, optimized, and innovated upon to create new assets, new commodities, and new productive and reproductive relationships of labor, value, and profit.[1] Biopolitics enables accumulation through dispossession, wherein producers are dispossessed of property rights over land, resources, and even the productive forces of their own bodies, by capital's accumulative power. While this is the bedrock of commodity capitalism (the transformation of natural resources into commodities to be sold at market), the distinguishing factor now is that life is essential to the productive, as opposed to exploitive, forces of late capitalism. Life is optimized and made to produce new forms of value. Michel Foucault points to how in capitalist societies capital and the human body are co-constitutive of biopolitics:

> [C]apitalism ... started by socializing its first object, the body, as a factor of productive force, as labor power. Society's control over individuals was accomplished not only through consciousness or ideology but also through the body and with the body. For capitalist society it was biopolitics, the biological, the somatic, the corporal that mattered more than anything else. The body is a biopolitical reality; medicine is the biopolitical strategy. (2003, p. 321)

Michael Hardt and Antonio Negri explain that biopolitics is a productive, rather than disciplinary, power in contemporary Western societies and, for our purposes in this chapter, US capitalist medicine (Hardt and Negri 2000, p. 27). The body, especially the human body, is the site of medical capitalism. Protected health data, taken from the bodies of patients who are dispossessed of any ownership claims over their data and its financial value, is standardized and instrumentalized through innovations made upon the data, through processes such as anonymization or big data analytics. These innovations unleash the data's accumulative forces that are harnessed by speculative medical capitalism. In what follows, I describe two innovations on private health data, de-identification and analytics, that make data useful and valuably productive.

The Privacy Promises and Market Values of Anonymization

As I explained in the previous chapter, the data standardization regulations under HIPAA, namely the Privacy Rule, the Security Rule, and the Omnibus Rule mandate that health providers and those organizations directly involved in some aspect of a patient's healthcare (such as a healthcare clearinghouse or a health insurer) must follow specific protocols to protect her information. The Security Rule regulates how digital information on a patient is appropriately secured (primarily through encryption), stored, and disclosed, by providing guidelines for data security standards and fining practices and hospitals when a breach occurs. The Omnibus Rule, passed in 2013, regulates the privacy and security of patient data, and includes third-party businesses in the protocol regime. Under this rule, both third parties and covered entities are liable for breaches.

The first innovation done to protected health data once it is collecte and abstracted from the bodies and lives of patients is de-identification. The promises of privacy pivot on the anonymization of health data. Privacy is big business in healthcare and it is through de-identification that a patient's data becomes a commodity. It is important to note here that there is a legal distinction between privacy and security. Data privacy is achieved through standardizing and securing personal health data. The HIPAA Privacy Rule mandates a "built-in" privacy function: the anonymization of health data. Before a patient's health data can move through the digitized data network, the individual record must be shorn of its identifying information, the 18 data points that comprise the protected health information (PHI) of a patient. This de-identification process is called the Safe Harbor method of data standardization, as outlined in §164.514(b) of the Privacy Rule. "Safe harboring" of protected health information must happen before the information is released to entities not directly involved in "healthcare operations," for example, before it is made into a database that is sold for medical and health research or for marketing purposes.

The PHI de-identification process is a crucial innovation that not only enables patient information to be mobilized though the network of disclosure but also enables it to be transformed into data assets that are bought and sold by third parties. The use of anonymized datasets—gleaned from sources as varied as the Centers for Disease Control (CDC), the Veterans Health Administration (VHA), electronic health records (EHR) software companies, and even from private data brokers—is, without a doubt, central to public health and medical research data analytics. Such analytics serve a vital public good, leading to beneficial outcomes for patients and the healthcare system on the whole. While data anonymization can and does serve this important purpose, it also provides financial benefits to private interests.

Let's take as an example prescription data, which is a key site of innovation and financial value for third-party companies. In an interview, Brogan Callahan, a data analyst who works for a subsidiary of the largest health informatics company in the world, IMS Health Inc., explained what happens to prescription data once it is received by a pharmacy. When a doctor writes a script for a patient, the prescription is electronically transferred through the doctor's EHR platform, faxed, or delivered on paper by the patient to a pharmacy. Once the prescription data is entered into the pharmacy's digital platform, the script is verified by a "switch" company, a third-party clearinghouse that checks the doctor's medical license, verifies that the doctor is authorized to prescribe the class of medication being ordered, validates the patient's information, and, for certain medications such as opioids, ascertains that a patient does not have multiple prescriptions filled at different pharmacies. All of these checks are done on the script's identifiable information. Once the prescription is validated as being legal and authentic by the switch company, the data is sent to the payer (the health insurer) for payment authorization, co-payment information, or claim rejection. All of this happens within a few minutes of receipt of the script. After all of the prescription fulfillment processes are complete, the script is de-identified by a third-party company that specializes in anonymizing health data (this process is often referred to as "data hygiene"). Josh Sims, a health informatics specialist who de-identifies health data for a large analytics corporation, explained to me that many who work in the data industry, hospitals, and health insurance companies consider identifiable health data to be something akin to nuclear waste: Everyone wants to get it off of their hands as quickly as possible because of the breach risks (and thus high penalties from Health and Human Services'[HHS] Office of Civil Rights). Once the data is cleaned of identifying information, it is ready to be sold to another third-party data analytics company, such as Callahan's company IMS Health Inc., which deals in a wide spectrum of health data, or Symphony Health Solutions, a company that focuses on prescription data. De-identified prescription data, along with data collected by the prescriber's electronic health records platform and other third-party datasets, is aggregated and packaged to become the data assets of these health informatics companies.

On the Internet, Everybody Knows You're a Patient

Although the de-identification of electronic health data might bring some a sense of security, this is nothing short of a collective delusion. The early years of the Internet promised that online anonymity would mean freedom and security. This is embodied in the iconic 1993 *New Yorker* cartoon depicting a dog in front of a computer, telling his dog-mate, "On the Internet, nobody knows that you're a dog." Looking back, this sense of security through anonymity seems downright naïve to us in the Age of Big Data (Steiner 1993). While I may feel better knowing that when my health record moves through the Internet it has been shorn of any identifying information that may link me to the record of my health and illness,

I really should not; nor should the health practitioners who are charged with stripping my record before it is released from their office. Even if they are complying with all regulations, it does not mean that they have secured my record and protected my privacy. As I described in Chapter 4, medical providers are doing the best they can, given the institutional constraints that they work within, and overwhelmingly, at least for the professionals that I interviewed, most healthcare workers endeavor to do what's best for their patients. All of us—patients, doctors, health records administrators, and chief privacy and HIPAA compliance officers—co-produce rituals of privacy, but in the end, these are magical-thinking practices.

While the de-identification of protected health information is one of those rituals that fulfills HIPAA's privacy and security requirements, a ritual that allows data to be mobilized, many privacy scholars have demonstrated that patients and their healthcare providers should not take much comfort in it—it is easy for data analysts to triangulate data and pinpoint individuals through even just a few data points. Privacy legal scholar Paul Ohm (2010) details how and why we should not trust the safe harboring of records, and warns that an individual can be re-identified with only few data points that appear to be completely anonymous, such as a zip code or a Netflix rating (Ohm 2010, p. 1705). There are several studies that demonstrate how easy it is to re-identify patients and directly connect them to protected health information. Latanya Sweeney, whose Data Map was described in the previous chapter, has conducted several re-identification studies on anonymized records, including her highly influential 1997 study that re-identified the hospitalization records of then-Massachusetts governor William Weld by using publicly available datasets and voter registration rolls. Her study ultimately changed safe harboring protocols (Barth-Jones 2012; Ohm 2010). Through her study of Weld's data, Sweeney demonstrated that for 87 percent of Americans, only three data points are needed to link a de-identified health record to a patient: zip code, sex, and birthdate (Ohm 2010, p. 1705).[2] After the passage of the 2003 Privacy Rule, Sweeney conducted another study of anonymized prescription data. In that study, the rate of re-identification under the Privacy Rule's safe harboring process was much higher than predicted: 6.1 percent rate of individuals were re-identified, compared to the predicted rate of 0.04 percent (Sweeney 2011, pp. 1–2). In another study, using a publicly available dataset of hospital admissions in the state of Washington, combined with information from news stories gleaned from LexisNexis, Sweeny was able to identify individual patients at a rate of 43 percent (Sweeney 2013, p. 9). Similarly, Yves-Alexandre de Montjoye and his co-authors demonstrate how easy it is to re-identify data from credit card records, which, as I discussed in Chapter 4, are used for payments for medical procedures. Using a dataset of 1.1 million credit card users who made purchases at 10,000 retailers in an Organisation for Economic Co-operation and Development (OECD) country, the researchers show that it only takes three data points—the date of the credit card transaction, the name of the vendor where the transaction was made, and the price of the transaction—to determine the cardholder's identity (de Montjoye et al. 2015). Finally, using only the metadata of research participants' phones ($N = 546$), Jonathan Mayer and Patrick Mutchler were able to pinpoint phone calls made on individual phones to health clinics and pharmacies, as well as online searches for medical information on heart ailments and HIV status. They were able to infer particular health conditions for each anonymous research subject in their study (Mayer and Mutchler 2014). As I described in Chapter 2, data brokers aggregate a combination of public data (Department of Motor Vehicles (DMV) records, voter registration) and private data (credit card transactions, browser cookies) into large datasets that can be sliced and funneled down to make inferences about an individual's consumer behavior for a variety of marketing purposes. In the case of health data, these methods are used to make inferences about an individual's health status, inferences, which are also used for marketing. As one list broker described to me, the current "hot spot" in the data marketing industry is health data.

Consider this common scenario: A patient has health insurance, and her doctor may bill her insurer for all or some of the procedures performed by herself or a nurse. Many health plans also include co-pays, which this patient pays for using her credit or debit card. This patient also uses funds from her flexible spending account (FSA), the tax-free savings account offered through her employer-sponsored healthcare plan and which comes with a VISA, MasterCard or Discover debit card which she must use to make payments from her FSA.[3] Although this patient's health data is de-identified and made "secure" under HIPAA before being transmitted to a third-party, the patient's debit or credit card data is not, regardless of whether the card is connected to a FSA or directly to the patient's bank account. For our patient's financial transaction to be authorized, certain identifying information will be transmitted from the clinic to a financial institution. Once this identifiable information is securely received by the bank or financing company, this data can be de-identified and leased or sold to any number of third parties, such as credit reporting bureaus or data brokerage firms.

Ownership Defines Us: The "Value-Add" of Anonymization and How Data Ownership Is Claimed

Resting data is dead data. For data to be useful within the network of disclosure, it must be reanimated and given new, productive life. Once the data are innovated upon by being de-identified, they become new objects: data assets. The data assets are then aggregated, analyzed, and distributed, producing value for those who claim ownership. US courts have consistently determined that data are owned by those who innovate on them, not those who produce them. Patients, and some health practitioners, may believe that patients own their health data or medical records, but, as many court cases have borne out, the law recognizes the property claims of innovators, not patients. There are parallels to these data ownership claims in other medical contexts, such as medical waste used in research and drug development. The most significant legal precedent for this logic is was provided by the California Supreme Court in *Moore v. Regents of the University of California, et al.* (1990). In this appellate case, plaintiff John Moore had been diagnosed with hairy-cell leukemia and had sought treatment from Dr. David Golde, an oncologist and medical researcher based at University of California, Los Angeles (UCLA). Golde removed Moore's spleen as part of his cancer treatment. In the process, he noticed that Moore's spleen was unusually productive of lymphokines, a protein essential to the immune system, which happens to be difficult to reproduce in large enough quantities for medical use. Golde recognized the market value of Moore's diseased spleen and, in collaboration with drug-maker Sandoz Pharmaceuticals, used Moore's "medical waste" to innovate a new therapeutic medicine for leukemia. At the time that Moore's spleen was removed, he was not informed that his tissues would be used to develop a new medicine, nor did he give his consent to this use of his tissue. Golde and Sandoz's innovation on Moore's cells was patented. The Court found that their innovation nullified any ownership claims that Moore may have felt were his over a piece of his body. Moore's spleen, and any resulting invention based upon it, became the bio-asset of Golde, UCLA, and Sandoz, who all made a lot of money from that asset. Moore lost his suit when the Supreme Court judges found in favor of the defendants, writing in the majority opinion that since Golde had performed necessary innovative labor to transform Moore's cells into a profitable commodity, the property rights cohere to the inventor, not to the original possessor of the tissue (Waldby and Mitchell 2006, pp. 88–93).

The network of disclosure mirrors this innovation-equals-ownership model for protected health information. Data ownership claims are made at several nodes within the network: by the hospital or doctor's office, by electronic health record vendors, by pharmacies that receive prescriptions, by health plans, and by third-party data aggregators and information services companies. The processes that make patient data secure under HIPAA are considered "innovations" upon those data. Consider the material and epistemic difference between locking a drawer and the HIPAA-compliant process that includes de-identifying thousands of patient records, encrypting data files through proprietary algorithms, and transmitting data through a networked software platform that is licensed to a hospital and stored on offsite, third-party servers; in digitized healthcare, securing data *is* innovation. In big data healthcare, data ownership and privacy rights shift away from the producers of data—patients, doctors, and nurses—to the innovators of data. In the bio-economic intellectual property regime, data is legally understood to be significantly transformed by the "inventive labor" of data security specialists and by data analytics, with profound consequences (Waldby and Mitchell 2006, p. 93).

As described in Chapter 2, many companies and organizations that are not in the business of aggregating and selling data as their core operations nevertheless will often turn to data that they possess as a potential revenue stream. The American Medical Association (AMA) maintains a database, the Physicians Masterfile, of more than 1.4 million licensed physicians across the USA, Puerto Rico, and other US territories. The list includes doctors regardless of their AMA affiliation, and includes identifiable information about each physician. The database is used for a variety of purposes, including verification and fraud detection. The AMA also sells this database to data brokers, primarily IMS Health Inc., which reportedly earns the association more than $40 million annually (Steinbrook 2006, p. 2747).[4] This database combines and triangulates prescription data that is purchased from retail pharmacies as well as from large prescription plans, such as Express Scripts Inc., which claim ownership over these prescription records.[5] IMS Health provides information on every script written by every physician in the AMA database to pharmaceutical makers for distribution to their sales forces. When news broke in 2013 that IMS

Health was purchasing the prescription behaviors of clinicians, many AMA physicians demanded an "opt-out" option. The AMA responded with the Physician Data Restriction Program, which enables members to declare that their prescription data can only be used for research purposes, and cannot be shared with drug marketing or sales forces (American Medical Association 2013). It should be noted that only about 4 percent of doctors use the opt-out option. Most doctors don't know about the option, or the fact that their prescription data is being sold in the first place (Thomas 2013). The opt-out only applies to the AMA data; there is no legal way that doctors can prevent pharmacies or health insurers from selling their prescription data (Thomas 2013). When doctors, patients and even state legislatures reacted against the practice of selling prescription data, especially without the consent of doctors or patients, the US Supreme Court favored data innovators in the 2011 case *Sorrell v. IMS Health Inc.* The majority of the court sided with data brokers' First Amendment right to sell prescription data as part of commercial speech (Boumil *et al.* 2012). While physicians are certainly an aggrieved group who rightly protest the sale of their prescription data, the traumas from these sales can be more acute for their patients, such as Marcy Campbell Krinsk, described in Chapter 1, who like me, was haunted by a marketing baby for a decade, after her prescription data had been sold after she purchased fertility drugs at a pharmacy in San Diego (Freudenheim 2009).

The data products provided by IMS Health are updated weekly in the databases of many pharmaceutical companies, according to Miranda Rosen, a pharmaceutical sales representative who specializes in drugs for pediatric epilepsy who I interviewed to learn more about how prescription data is used by third parties, such as drug companies. Rosen uses this data in her regular sales visits that she makes to the two hundred physicians in her "portfolio," and the prescribing information is essential to how she targets her marketing messages to doctors.

Brogan Callahan, the data analyst mentioned earlier in the chapter, explains that while there can be many ownership claims made over health data, courts continuously recognize innovators, like IMS Health or pharmacies, as owning health data:

> [Health data] can be owned, really, by multiple entities. ... If you look at pure ownership, in terms of if you licensed it, and then improved it or did something with the information, applied some sort of analytical overlay, and then used it internally, then that is inherently different than what was

> initially received. It's sort of like what we refer to in our industry as a value-added re-seller. ... If I license data to you, I license it, I don't sell it, and if you then want to turn around and license it to somebody else, you have to do something to it: you have to put it in a product that provides different types of information. ... [I]f you collect information from a public domain and then aggregate it all together, and then license it to somebody else, then that's a product that you've just created, based on a lot of disparate pieces of information. That, in my eyes, would be ownership, but then you talk to the person who the data is referencing, and they might say, 'That's my information, and it's mine, and you can't do anything with it,' but yet it's publicly available, so, then, who's right?

It is significant how Callahan characterizes personal data collected from the public domain, as what is "public" is a fungible concept, at least in the eyes of data brokers. It is through this fungibility of public and private information that data commodities are made and mobilized. Those working to protect the data of patients, especially in regard to ownership and profitability, are keenly aware of this as well. In May 2013, the Executive Office of Management and Budget (OMB) released a memorandum titled "Open Data Policy—Managing Information as an Asset" to the heads of all federal departments. It outlined Executive Order of May 9, 2013 requiring government data to be "machine readable" and easily accessible by the public (Burwell *et al.* 2013). The memorandum's opening paragraph reflects the common boosterism rhetoric that links big data to economic prosperity: "Making information resources accessible, discoverable, and usable by the public can help fuel entrepreneurship, innovation, and scientific discovery—all of which improve Americans' lives and contribute significantly to job creation" (Burwell et al. 2013, p. 1). The executive order's Open Data mandate stated that all data produced by taxpayer funds should be considered "owned" by the public, and therefore, should be publicly available online. One regulator at the Veterans Health Administration (VHA) who was charged with protecting the health data of those veterans who receive VHA healthcare and those who participate in VHA medical research was concerned that the Open Data mandate would result in a public data free-for-all for private enterprise. He knew that data brokers scrape federal websites for public data and commodify it. So in response to the Open Data mandate, the VHA put in place a data management plan that follows the OMB's mandate but respects the data ownership rights of veterans by meeting the bare minimum of the mandate and severely restricting the use and access of veteran health data (Puglisi 2015).

Possession Plus Innovation Equals Ownership

Data privacy, security, and ownership take on significantly different meanings in digital forms. Josh Sims, the bioinformatics analyst introduced in Chapter 2, describes this difference as one where the innovations in data security cannot keep up with the algorithms that are invented to disclose and re-identify health data. The Health Information Technology for Economic and Clinical Health (HITECH) Act (introduced in Chapter 4) and the Affordable Care Act (111th Congress 2010) both mandate health practice changes that use either financial incentives or non-compliance penalties to induce patients to disclose their health information. Primarily, the HITECH Act mandates that all US health providers demonstrate "meaningful use" of electronic health records (EHR) for all of their patients. The Act also regulates the security of EHRs. Between 2011 and 2014, healthcare providers received financial incentives to adopt the use of health records software and transfer all of their records to electronic systems. In 2015, those rewards converted to punishments in the form of reductions in Medicare reimbursements for non- or slow-adopters (Athena Health Inc. 2009). Prior to the 2015 deadline, practices could use the financial incentives to help offset the costs of EHR implementation. The EHR requirements have not been as burdensome for larger health systems as they have for mid-sized and smaller systems and practices. The cost of purchasing and maintaining software, servers, and other equipment, as well as the diverted labor and compliance consulting, was quite steep for some smaller practices, some of which chose to close down rather than be compliant with HITECH.

Since it was folded into the larger stimulus package to reverse the 2008 economic crisis, the HITECH Act was a boon for certain sectors of healthcare industry. One of the most obvious beneficiaries of this legislation is the EHR industry, as companies like Epic Systems Corporation and Allscripts Healthcare Solutions Inc. realized a ready-made market (Perna 2012; SK&A 2015). In 2015, the global EHR software market exceeded $23 billion, and within the USA, the market is dominated by a handful of vendors (Monegain 2014; SK&A 2015). As far back as 1995, before HIPAA was finalized, there was concern among legislators over the purchase of patient data contained within electronic health records, when the EHR industry was in its infancy, by IMS Health Inc. or data broker and credit bureau, Equifax Inc. (Kolata 1995).

In an interview, Amelia Cook, the emergency-room nurse that we met in the previous chapter, she described the process of moving from paper to digital records at her hospital. Cook has worked as an emergency pediatric nurse at the same hospital for 13 years, and during that entire time she has seen patient health records move from paper to digital files. This transfer has accelerated in the last six years, to the point where her hospital's recordkeeping is now almost fully electronic. As one can imagine, such a migration from paper to electronic records is much more of a challenge for small, community hospitals and family practices than for the large and powerful healthcare system that Cook works for.

Under HITECH, a patient cannot "opt-out" of digital records, nor can they ask for their medical and health information to be stored on paper. Furthermore, many EHR software companies compel physicians to either sell or hand over patient data to the software vendor through their data use agreements. These agreements often cede ownership of de-identified patient data to the EHR vendor, especially those vendors that offer "free" cloud-based platforms. In many ways, these digital health records platforms are much like Facebook in that all of the information input through the software becomes the property of the vendor. For example, the cloud-based EHR vendor, Practice Fusion, offers healthcare systems a freeware version of their web-based platform. The freeware version actually does come with a price tag: There are advertisements within the software, similar to those in Facebook or Gmail, and through the user agreements, practices agree to share the data within the platform with Practice Fusion, including the data collected when a doctor or nurse clicks on an in-platform ad (Pottenger 2010).[6] Practice Fusion assuredly explains in their promotional literature for the product that these data are HIPAA-compliant and anonymized (Pottenger 2010, p. 3). The data contained within a doctor or nurse's clicking behavior, just like in the case of Facebook, becomes the property of Practice Fusion, who can sell it to other third parties. This means that when patient discloses her information to her doctor, and he enters it into her electronic health record, this data no longer is owned by the patient whose body and health produced the data, nor by the doctor who purchased the software license and consulted with the patient to input the data. Instead, it is owned by a third party. Again, the data innovator has ownership, not the data producer.

Under the Omnibus Rule, a patient does have the right to request and receive her health record, either printed or in a digital format, from her doctor. In my research for this book, I requested my full medical record from the fertility clinic, and for a charge of $67.50 plus tax, I was sent a paper copy—a 186-page pile of paper. Within the copy, not only was there a record of every visit, every lab (but no ultrasound images), and every phone call, but also all of the data collected during my participation in the clinical trial. In addition to being able to access a printed copy of her record, a patient also has a right to gain online access to portions of her health record, as long as she is verified and registered through her doctor's web-based system. Despite a patient's right to access her health record, she does not own her data, as she ceded her ownership rights through her health disclosures to her doctor. In my interviews with health practitioners, only one person, a surgeon and the oldest person to participate in interviews, asserted that a patient owns her record. No other doctor or nurse that I interviewed made such a claim. Most either were unsure or flatly stated that while they can have access to their medical records, patients do not own them; those ownership rights belong to the health practice. Only Callahan, the data analyst, claimed that third-party innovators of health data own the record.

This point was underlined in my interview with Brianna Herve, a clinical informatics specialist working in an urban hospital system. During our discussion about the EHR platforms that are used within her hospital, which are her specialty, she mentioned that the hospital is working toward implementing a web-based system that allows patients to access their EHR. This has implications for data ownership, privacy, and control. When asked who owns a patient's data, Brianna said hesitantly and somewhat apologetically:

> If you asked me I would say we would like, in a perfect world, for the patient to own the data. Because it's their data. In my experience, if a patient finds something in their chart that they don't agree with or they don't like, it is nearly impossible to get it removed. I wouldn't say that we're at that perfect level yet.

In the network of disclosure, data ownership is granted, time and again, to those who are in possession of the information and those who innovate upon the data, either through de-identification or analytics. Similarly, as Brogan Callahan, the health data analyst, boiled down data ownership claims made by data brokers on patient records, that "[i]t's similar to the 'who owns a genetic code' [question]. Does the company own the gene sequence that they took from people during some unrelated procedure, or does it belong to the person who it came from?" Despite the claim made by healthcare practitioners, like Brianna, that patients do indeed own their data and their health record, legislation, court cases, and industry practices do not bear this out. Patients and even their doctors, simply do not own their health data.

Notes

1. Several scholars have developed rich and engaging scholarship on biocapital, which takes up where Foucault left off with biopolitics to consider the production of "biovalue," "bio-assets," "biolabor," and new forms of capitalist speculation and promissory capital based on genomics, reproductive technologies, and other life sciences. See, for example, Rose's *The Politics of Life Itself* (2007); Melinda Cooper's and Catherine Waldby's work on biolabor and surplus biovalue in fertility medicine (Cooper and Waldby 2014; Waldby and Cooper 2010), and Kaushik Sunder Rajan's work on genomics, biospeculation, and biocapitalism (Rajan 2005, 2006).
2. Ohm (2010) observes that some scholars, such as Phillipe Golle, replicated Sweeney's original experiment but could not produce the same results of 87 percent. However, Golle's findings still showed that 63 percent of the population could be uniquely identified.
3. Retail and investment banks, such as Bank of America, offer services directly to employers to implement and manage the FSA benefit at their workplaces. See, for example, Bank of America's website for such services: http://healthaccounts.bankofamerica.com.
4. Despite my best efforts to retrieve a more up-to-date Physicians Masterfile revenue figure, including downloading the AMA's most recently available IRS 990 return, I was unable to find it. Steinbrook's figure was gleaned from the AMA's 2005 Annual Report, a document that is only available to members.
5. In *Steinberg v. CVS Caremark Corp.* a civil lawsuit brought to the District Court of Pennsylvania in 2012, plaintiffs sued the retail pharmacy for their unauthorized sale of patient prescription data. The Court dismissed the case, in part due to the pharmacy's data ownership claims: CVS argued that the company de-identifies and aggregates prescription data before selling it to pharmaceutical companies (*Arthur Steinberg, et al. v. CVS Caremark Corporation, et al.* 2012).
6. In a company white paper that describes the revenue model for its freeware version of Practice Fusion, the author notes that "...by embedding advertisements in a banner at the bottom of its electronic medical record system and by selling anonymized patient and doctor data from its system to third parties, maintaining HIPAA compliance along the way [sic]. Practice Fusion also gives physicians the option to operate an ad-free electronic medical record system for $250 per month. However, as expected, most physicians choose to run the advertisement-based model" (Pottenger 2010, p. 3).

References

111th Congress. 2010. *Patient Protection and Affordable Care Act (ACA)*. 42 USC 18001.

Almeling, Rene. 2011. *Sex Cells: The Medical Market for Eggs and Sperm*. Berkeley: University of California Press.

American Medical Association. 2013. *AMA Program Helps Protect Doctor Prescribing Information: Q & A with American Medical Association Board of Trustees Member Jeremy A. Lazarus, MD*. Chicago: American Medical Association. http://www.ama-assn.org/ama1/pub/upload/mm/371/pdrp_qa_final.pdf.

Arthur Steinberg, et al. v. CVS Caremark Corporation, et al. 2012, 899 F.Supp.2d 331. 2012. Pennsylvania: United States District Court, Eastern District.

Athena Health Inc. 2009. "A Summary of the HITECH Act." White Paper. Watertown, MA: Athena Health.

Barth-Jones, Daniel C. 2012. "The 'Re-Identification' of Governor William Weld's Medical Information: A Critical Re-Examination of Health Data Identification Risks and Privacy Protections, Then and Now." Pre-Publication Working Paper. Epidemiology, Mailman School of Public Health, Columbia University. http://ssrn.com/abstract=2076397.

Boumil, Marcia M., Kaitlyn Dunn, Nancy Ryan, and Katrina Clearwater. 2012. "Prescription Data Mining, Medical Privacy and the First Amendment: The U.S. Supreme Court in Sorrell v. IMS Health Inc." *Annals of Health Law* 21 (2): 447–91.

Burwell, Sylvia M., Steven VanRoekel, Todd Park, and Dominic J. Mancini. 2013. "M-13-13 Memorandum for the Heads of Executive Departments and Agencies; Subject: Open Data Policy-Managing Information as an Asset." Memorandum, May 9.

Cooper, Melinda, and Catherine Waldby. 2014. *Clinical Labor: Tissue Donors and Research Subjects in the Bioeconomy*. Durham, NC: Duke University Press.

de Montjoye, Yves-Alexandre, Laura Radaelli, Vivek Kumar Singh, and Alex "Sandy" Pentland. 2015. "Unique in the Shopping Mall: On the Reidentifiability of Credit Card Metadata." *Science* 347 (6221): 536–39.

Foucault, Michel. 2003. "The Birth of Social Medicine." In *The Essential Foucault: The Essential Works of Foucault 1954-1984*, edited by Paul Rabinow and Nikolas Rose, 319–37. New York: New Press.

Freudenheim, Milt. 2009. "And You Thought a Prescription Was Private." *The New York Times*, August 9, sec. Business, BU1.

Hardt, Michael, and Antonio Negri. 2000. *Empire*. Cambridge, MA: Harvard University Press.

Kolata, Gina. 1995. "When Patients' Records Are Commodities for Sale." *New York Times*, November 15, C14.

Lemke, Thomas. 2011. *Biopolitics*. New York: New York University Press.

Mayer, Jonathan, and Patrick Mutchler. 2014. "MetaPhone: The Sensitivity of Telephone Metadata." *Web Policy*, March 12. Accessed January 9, 2016. http://webpolicy.org/2014/03/12/metaphone-the-sensitivity-of-telephone-metadata.

Monegain, Bernie. 2014. "EMR Market Surpasses $23 Billion." *HealthcareITnews.com*, April 29. Accessed January 9, 2016. http://www.healthcareitnews.com/news/emr-market-surpasses-23-billion.

Moore v. Regents of University of California, 271 Cal.Rptr. 146 51 Cal.3d 120 (Supreme Court of California 1990).

Ohm, Paul. 2010. "Broken Promises of Privacy: Responding to the Surprising Failure of Anonymization." *UCLA Law Review* 57 (6): 1701–77.

Pateman, Carole. 2002. "Self-Ownership and Property in the Person: Democratization and a Tale of Two Concepts." *Journal of Political Philosophy* 10 (1): 20–53.

Perna, Gabriel. 2012. "EMR Market Dominated by Top Six Companies." *Healthcare Informatics*, March 23. Accessed January 9, 2016. http://www.healthcare-informatics.com/print/news-item/emr-market-dominated-top-six-companies.

Phillips, Anne. 2013. *Our Bodies, Whose Property?* Princeton, NJ: Princeton University Press.

Pottenger, Brent. 2010. "'Freeconomics' in Health Care: Practice Fusion and the Future of Free, Web-Based Health Information Systems." White Paper. San Francisco, CA: Practice Fusion. http://www.practicefusion.com/whitepapers/business-model-freeconomics/.

Puglisi, Tom. 2015. *Policy and Implementation Plan for Public Access to Scientific Publications and Digital Data from Research Funded by the Department of Veterans Affairs.* Data Management Plan. Washington, DC: VHA Office of Research Oversight. http://www.va.gov/ORO/Docs/Guidance/VA_RSCH_DATA_ACCESS_PLAN_07_23_2015.pdf.

Radin, Margaret Jane. 1996. *Contested Commodities: The Trouble with Trade in Sex, Children, Body Parts, and Other Things.* Cambridge, MA: Harvard University Press.

Rajan, Kaushik Sunder. 2005. "Subjects of Speculation: Emergent Life Sciences and Market Logics in the United States and India." *American Anthropologist* 107 (1): 19–30.

———. 2006. *Biocapital: The Constitution of Postgenomic Life.* Durham, NC: Duke University Press.

Rose, Nikolas. 2007. *The Politics of Life Itself: Biomedicine, Power, and Subjectivity in the Twenty-First Century.* Princeton, NJ: Princeton University Press.

Scheper-Hughes, Nancy. 2001. "Bodies for Sale: Whole or in Parts." *Body & Society* 7 (2–3): 1–8.

SK&A. 2015. *Physician Office Usage of Electronic Health Records Software.* Irvine, CA: SK&A.

Steinbrook, Robert. 2006. "For Sale: Physicians' Prescribing Data." *New England Journal of Medicine* 354 (26): 2745–47.

Steiner, Peter. 1993. *On the Internet, Nobody Knows You're a Dog*. Cartoon. New Yorker Collection/Cartoon Bank.

Sweeney, Latanya. 2011. "Patient Identifiability in Pharmaceutical Marketing Data." Data Privacy Lab Working Paper 1015. Cambridge, UK. http://dataprivacylab.org/projects/identifiability/pharma1.html

———. 2013. "Matching Known Patients to Health Records in Washington State Data." White Paper 1089-1. Cambridge, MA: Data Lab, Harvard University.

Thomas, Katie. 2013. "Data Trove on Doctors Guides Drug Company Pitches." *New York Times*, May 17, sec. Business Day, B1.

Waldby, Catherine, and Melinda Cooper. 2010. "From Reproductive Work to Regenerative Labour: The Female Body and the Stem Cell Industries." *Feminist Theory* 11 (1): 3–22.

Waldby, Catherine, and Robert Mitchell. 2006. *Tissue Economies: Blood, Organs, and Cell Lines in Late Capitalism*. Durham, NC: Duke University Press.

CHAPTER 6

The Uncanny Lives of Data Commodities

Comrades

As I lay prone, naked from the waist down and my feet in stirrups, with the speculum protruding from my vagina, I strained under the discomfort of my very full bladder as it pressed into my lower abdomen, demanding to be emptied. I had been directed by the nurse assisting in the embryo transfer to drink plenty of fluids because they needed my bladder to be full so that when the embryologist made the embryo transfer, my bladder would appear on the ultrasound's monitor as a white, glowing blob. This would provide a good, visual contrast for her to see the air bubble containing the two embryos as it traveled out of the catheter and into my uterus. During that moment, I too would be able to "see" my embryos for a moment before they nestled into the infinite blackness of the screen's pixels.

My doctor was not on duty that day. Reproductive biology works on its own timing and thus, my artificial cycle was out-of-sync with the clinic's duty schedule, despite their efforts to engineer my body's hormonal rhythm to align with the work cycle of the clinic. Although my usual doctor was Dr. Gaunkar, that day there was a new doctor on call sitting next to me, someone I had never met before. As we waited for the embryologist to come into the operating room to make the transfer, we traded nods and small talk. He smiled politely and remained seated, close to my head, but he still looked down to meet my gaze, as I was lying with my pelvis slightly raised. That position would afford the clinicians performing the

M.F.E. Ebeling, *Healthcare and Big Data*,
DOI 10.1057/978-1-137-50221-6_6

transfer optimum access both physically and visually to my vagina, the os of my cervix, and uterus.

"Hi, I'm Dr. Phillips, Dr. Gaonkar is not on duty today, so I'm going to oversee the transfer for her," he said and offered his hand, reaching across the bed and the green sheet covering my chest. My breasts were heavy and tender under the influence of all of the synthetic hormones coursing through my veins.

I shook his hand.

"Oh, thanks for helping today," was about all I could muster over the pounding of my bladder, which was made more intense by the speculum sticking out of me. I offered a small smile, trying to convey a complexity of meaning: It was an expression that I hoped indicated I was a compliant patient but also one that suggested to him that I was very aware of the awkwardness of the situation. After all, I was lying below him, him fully dressed, me half naked, with my vagina and cervix propped up under the glare of the examination lights.

"You're participating in the clinical trial that Dr. Gaonkar is heading up?" he asked. I wasn't sure he received the intended meaning of my smile.

"Yeah, we are really happy to be able to participate, because this is our last chance to try and have a baby. We couldn't afford any more IVF [in vitro fertilization]." After eight unsuccessful cycles of intrauterine insemination, and three rounds of IVF, one in which I failed to produce enough ripened eggs, one that resulted in a miscarriage, and one in which I didn't get pregnant at all, this Phase III clinical trial testing the effectiveness of an IVF drug was our last-ditch effort to try and produce a child with assisted reproductive technologies.

Dr. Phillips gently nodded and pursed his lips in understanding.

"So, what do you do?" Dr. Phillips asked in a friendly, small talk, chatty sort of way. He seemed somewhat oblivious to my discomfort, but it did occur to me that this was his regular "workday" experience: a woman splayed, on display, and dying to pee.

"Well, I'm a sociologist. In fact, some of what I study is science and medicine." I replied, with a wry, little grin that I hoped was just suggestive enough to Dr. Phillips that he would keep on his toes that morning because it was quite possible that I was studying him and the clinic.

"Ah, interesting," he said and, for an instant his face hardened, almost imperceptibly. After a beat he added, "You see all of this?"

He gestured around the room at the ultrasound machine with the vaginal probe, the magic wand that is inserted to see what is happening deep inside my uterus, the cabinets filled with syringes and sponges, the computer screen in the corner displaying my electronic health record (EHR). Finally, he turned his eyes back to land on me, as I lay on the gurney. "This is all capitalism."

I perked up and raised myself a bit on my elbows, despite my bladder. How I wished I had my notebook and voice recorder right now!

From there, Dr. Phillips cited numerous succinct and clipped examples to relay his critical analysis of the political economy of global reproductive biocapitalism, which produces subjects, commodities, and objects that are enmeshed in complex, dialogic relationships (Rajan 2006). He illustrated the global production and trade in highly lucrative synthetic hormones through the story of the development of follicle stimulating hormone (FSH), an essential drug used in assisted reproduction. He told me that hormonal production on a mass scale was made possible by postmenopausal nuns living in convents across Italy who collected their morning urine—voluntarily and without remuneration—and donated it to the Vatican-invested pharmaceutical manufacturer EMD Serono, the inventor of the synthetic FSH hormone GONAL-F (Dichek 2011).[1] He deftly connected those elderly nuns' bodies and their biolabor to pregnant horses in North America that are kept in continuous breeding cycles so that people can collect and synthesize estrogens from their urine for the large-scale manufacture of synthetic estrogens such as PREMARIN ("*Pre*gnant *Mar*es' Ur*in*e") for use in humans, and to the global market for oocytes often sourced from women who live lives of economic and political precariousness (Waldby and Cooper 2010).[2] In fact, he told me, for an additional $800 paid to the clinic, I could review the clinic's catalogue of available egg "donors" or the adoptable embryos "left over" from other couples' successful IVF cycles. I could choose eggs drawn from women who, despite their self-descriptions of the altruistic motives for donating their eggs to strangers, could not help but be swayed by the $10,000 they would be paid. He explained that innovations in medical science and technologies are often impossible without the work done within the university hospital setting, much like the one that we both found ourselves in, an institution supported by a mix of public and private investment. Through his gaze and words, he connected all of this back to patients like myself: I was part of and produced by this global, fleshy network of biocommodities. So was Dr. Phillips. We are all a part of it, enmeshed in it.

Could Dr. Phillips be reading the same books that I was during his time off from the clinic? What he was describing, presumably born out of his own embedded experiences within the reproductive medicine industry, resonated closely with the scholarship of social scientists and philosophers who study the biomedical and life sciences as outsiders. In his groundbreaking book on the global genomics industry, anthropologist Kaushik S. Rajan (2006) develops a theory of biocapitalism, and he richly describes the global circuits of genomic "currencies"—the financial investment funds that focus on life science start-ups, or on biological materials such as cell lines and engineered life forms like Onco Mouse. Rajan and other scholars, such as Catherine Waldby and Nikolas Rose, whose work was introduced in previous chapters, argue that these commodities contain new forms of value: biovalue (Rajan 2006, p. 43; Waldby and Mitchell 2006; Rose 2007). Philosopher and queer-feminist theorist Paul Preciado similarly conceptualizes the global hormonal circuits that Dr. Phillips described to me, as cybercommunication within the "pharmacopornographic era," or the epoch of techno-biopower that connects human and non-human bodies, through which a pharmaco-technical subjectivity is produced by *live* capital, or biocapitalism (Preciado 2013; Haraway 1997, 2008). Preciado writes, "pharmacopornographic biocapitalism does not produce things. It produces movable ideas, living organs, symbols, desires, chemical reactions, and affects. … [T]here are no objects to produce; it's a matter of inventing a subject and producing it on a global scale" (2013, loc 587). In his book *Testo Junkie* (2013), Preciado documents his use of testosterone during his time of experimentation with the fluidness of gender embodiment. Through his experiential narrative, he expands Rajan's concept of the biocapital circuit of commodities to include the immaterial qualities of biocommodities, including affect, kinship, and intellectual properties. These immaterial qualities fuel and lubricate the network that ultimately produces subjects of biocapital, and not merely biocommodities alone. Biocapitalism produces mobile subjects and objects that circulate. Preciado notes that Foucault's architectural and epistemic structural subjects of biopower cannot account for the flows of hormonal gender normativity, including the desire to make babies with the hormones, oocytes, spermatozoa, and uteri of others. Preciado firmly situates himself as a pharmacopornographic subject within global biocapital each time he (as Beatriz) rubs himself serendipitously with self-administered testosterone. He does this as an act of bioterrorism and defiance, as a ritual of mourning, and as an experimental re-engineering and re-inventing of the gendered body. Similarly, I was also a biocapital subject with each shot of FSH and progesterone that I injected into my legs and stomach (Preciado 2013; Thompson 1999).[3] And Dr. Phillips told me as much as well.

Dr. Phillips, I detected, or perhaps I projected this upon him, was not pleased with the global biocapital-pharmacological system that he found himself entangled in alongside his patients, colleagues, and myriad unnamed and unknown others. That day at the clinic, I was not able to engage him further on the topic, as the embryologist, covered in sterile paper scrubs and mask, and delicately holding the long, thin catheter containing my three-day-old, eight-celled embryos, interrupted our conversation. She crouched down close to my vagina, and gently inserted the catheter into the frowning os of my cervix, which lost its roundness when I gave birth to my daughter years ago. The three of us, with our heads turned toward the black, white, and gray screen watched intently as Dr. Phillips rubbed my lower belly with the ultrasound's wand.

"There! You see it?" With his free hand, Dr. Phillips lightly touched the screen. The gray pixels momentarily lightened as the embryonic bubbles bobbed and then faded into the darkness.

Dr. Phillips sat silently next to me still watching the screen. I fantasize that I had a covert, insider anti-biocapitalist comrade and saboteur sitting next to me through the two minutes of the procedure. Like a night-terror apparition that dissolves in the morning light, after the transfer was complete, I never saw Dr. Phillips again.

My Body as Data Subject-Object of Biocapital

I enrolled in the randomized, double-blind controlled clinical trial PURSUE hoping to become pregnant and to give birth to a live baby. The trial was sponsored by the pharmaceutical giant Schering-Plough,[4] and tested corifollitropin alfa, a follicular stimulant. I did not participate in the clinical trial selflessly, using my body and the data that it produces to help others. I used my body because I wanted to help myself, as many other patients do who participate in randomized trials as part of their clinical care. I balanced the chance of receiving the placebo against receiving treatment that I could no longer afford (Timmermans 2010). I still had to pay for some trial procedures out of pocket (I put them on my credit card), such as "assisted hatching," where my fertilized eggs were hatched with chemicals or a laser so that the embryonic cells could more easily grow and reproduce in vitro. While my hope was partially realized—I did get pregnant from that trial—the pregnancy did not result in a living, breathing baby. Instead it produced a ghostly marketing baby.

All of the data that my body produced for the trial, as well as all of the data from my past experiences of trying to get pregnant and give birth through reproductive technologies, lives on as a data commodity, a biocommodity, a data *thing* activated by lively capital (Haraway 2008, pp. 45–46). Data concerning my body's chemical-physiological responses to the study drug were carefully collected by the clinic's research nurses, entered into an electronic record, and algorithmically anonymized by numerical code. The data was handed back to Schering-Plough, but it was also entered into the electronic medical record kept by the clinic—which was attached to my identity. During my participation in the trial, I carefully recorded data about myself in a study log (a paper notebook) that was given to me by the head research nurse. All of these data were also entered into my anonymized record. Finally, the results of this medical procedure—the fact that I did indeed get pregnant because of IVF and the clinical trial—became marketing and promotional data used by Schering-Plough to demonstrate the efficacy of the study drug. That material comprised part of the pharmaceutical company's New Drug Application (NDA) to the US Food and Drug Administration (FDA). Certainly as well, my pregnancy was used to promote the clinic. After all, at my first appointment, Dr. Gaonkar showed me a table of the clinic's pregnancy and live birth rates, as a way of "selling" the clinic to me as a new patient.

My data was transformed into a commodity through the innovations made upon it and through its transfer from the clinic to the pharmaceutical company, which, as I described in Chapter 5, legally owns my data. With this transformation, data's exchange value is realized and captured. The bio-based data commodity is imbued with a "phantom-like objectivity" that takes on a power and agency of its own (Marx 1976, vol. 1, p. 128). Social conditions—the clinical trial, the fact that I was a patient, the global reproductive medicine industry, the big data industry—help construct the data commodity. There is an aura that surrounds the data commodity that is invisible but eerily, and ever, present. It is now quite common to hear someone say that she is "creeped out" when the online ads in her browser seem to "know" that she has a certain diagnosis. In a 2015 *Bloomberg News* article about "matchbacks," a marketing technique that can identify web users through matching their prescription data with their browsers to "serve" them customized ads, one patient interviewed said, "[i]t's this uncanny sense of, is this computer reading my mind? It's almost as if the computer pops up the ad even before the thought pops in your head" (Robertson and Pettypiece 2014). That uncanniness is the data commodity's aura shining through the computer screen.

Market logics suffuse the anonymization, repackaging, and abstraction of health data (Rajan 2006, p. 42). This is the value of the thing and through this transmutation, the data goes on to live a life of its own in the databases of the clinic, the pharmaceutical company sponsoring the drug study, and, quite possibly, health informatics analysts or medical researchers unconnected to the clinical trial. Clearly, at least some of my medical data and my protected health information, sourced from my credit card transactions and prescription data, was sold to data brokers who combined it with my online searches about assisted reproduction, as I described in Chapter 5. Out of these sociotechnical confluences, these data things are born and take on lives of their own.

The Data Commodity Comes to Haunt Me

Marx recognized that capital's objects, commodities, are things that are bruised by the traumas that go into their making: "Capital [and commodities] comes [into the world] dripping from head to toe, from every pore, of blood and dirt" (Marx 1976, vol. 1, p. 926, my additions in brackets). What are data commodities? How do they haunt us? How are they bruised and bloodied by trauma? Data commodities are "things" that are both material and immaterial. These objects are both made by us and precede us. Data things are deep and shallow; they are familiar and strange. Data things, like my marketing baby data revenant, are uncanny (Freud 2003). Data things are both subjects and objects; they have agency and power. In the Age of Big Data, we are made into data things; we are both subjects and objects, as I showed in Chapters 2 and 5. Data things often collapse into a "data image" that looks a lot like data phrenology, or what some media theorists call an algorithmic identity, where data brokers infer and construct our identities that I mentioned in Chapter 2. In the process, data make us legible and marketable (Cheney-Lippold 2011; Markham 2013). As I have already shown, for data brokers as well as for the network of disclosure, we *are* commodities and at the same time, data commodities are made *of* us and return to confront us in new forms, like in the shape of a FICO credit score. Furthermore, these data commodities are marked by the violence that went into their making. Daniel Solove describes the violence of databases and the data commodities that arise from them:

> [T]he problem with databases and the practices currently associated with them is that they disempower people. They make people vulnerable by stripping them of control over their personal information. There is no diabolical motive or secret plan for domination: rather there is a web of thoughtless decisions made by low-level bureaucrats, standardized policies, rigid routines, and a way of relating to individuals and their information that often becomes indifferent to their welfare. (Solove 2006, p. 41)

Data commodities are immaterial things that, in the process of rematerialization, can cause real, material harm. They are both mundane and horrific.

Cultural anthropologists understand things as cultural artifacts, as objects, that embody the social relations that went into making them. As such, things have both a material form and a ghostly aura. Things can embody a society's aspirations and goals, or index a culture's demons, like a straw man or effigy that is burnt and destroyed to symbolically rid the culture of an undesired value or fear (Brown 2001). Things are hollow and covered with a shell, or a skin, of the "real." But if you scratch the surface, there is a void. We make things. Things make us as well. This making is always violent, and the dispossession we undergo is traumatizing.

Do data subjects make data things, as with Victor Frankenstein and his Creature? Or is the relationship more ambivalent? Are data things asserting themselves as active agents in a particular subject-object relation (Brown 2001, p. 4)? Are data things, like all commodities, projections of our desires? A data thing that thinks and that speaks. My marketing baby is a data thing that visits me through marketing materials, knocks at my door and asks to be let in. At times, I have welcomed this phantom. At times, there is something reassuring in the thought that I do indeed have a baby, somewhere, even if it is comprised of crystals, electrons, and beams of flashing lights, and lives a highly distributed life across the databases of untold data brokers.

My marketing baby, the embodiment of my health and consumer data, was summoned from disparate databases by Experian's patented algorithm, reassembled into a mailing list that was sold to American List Counsel Inc., and transported into their "*Newborn Network*" database (Chamberlain *et al.* 2015; Engel and Kigler 2013). In this chapter, I use my marketing baby to consider how health data is rematerialized and reanimated into a data commodity or a data thing. I demonstrate how information about our most intimate traumas and losses, our bodies rendered legible through data by capitalist medicine, can be commodified. Rajan observes that within biocapitalism, the bio-based commodity fetish—and I consider my marketing baby to be a bio-derived data commodity—does not result from a process of alienation, with "the assumption of a transcendental thing-in-itself," but rather from a process of interpellation, where the "thing" hails the subject (the patient) directly (2006, p. 168; Althusser 2001). Health data commodities are not entirely alienated from the patient, even though the patient may be dispossessed of their data and no longer recognize the value of what they produced. Every time that my marketing baby rings my doorbell, calls me up on the phone, appears in places such as *American Baby* magazine, shows up in my Facebook feed, asks me to reply to an unsolicited email, and implores me to buy it things, it increases its life as a data commodity and multiplies the marketing value of my health data.

My marketing baby has a birth month (March 2011), a home, and even a class identity, which I discuss in the next chapter. However, my marketing baby does not have a name, and its gender and racial identity may be left to speculation, inferred by the data brokers who were the midwives at my marketing baby's birth. How do I know that my marketing baby is living a life of its own? Because it comes to visit me with flesh of paper and ink. I have seen it, touched it, and held it.

I Am Not a Baby

In late March 2011, I received a piece of direct marketing mail, which I sketched into my detective's notebook as another bit of evidence (Fig. 6.1). When it arrived, I was carrying my dead fetus in my uterus, waiting for the dilation and curettage procedure to be done by Dr. Gaonkar. Yes, it is possible to be "not quite pregnant" and to house death within one's living body. For two agonizing weeks I was full of death. Figure 6.1 is a drawing that depicts a piece of evidence that comprises my marketing baby's "body": a direct marketing envelope from Enfamil, addressed to me, which contains coupons and information about the Enfamil product line of breast milk substitutes. This envelope was one small part of the entire "body of evidence" that I collected as "proof" that my marketing baby was alive and being summoned by data marketers out of data warehouses.

The envelope was printed with the image of a swaddled newborn, and the text below declares in bold Helvetica font, "I am not a baby. I am

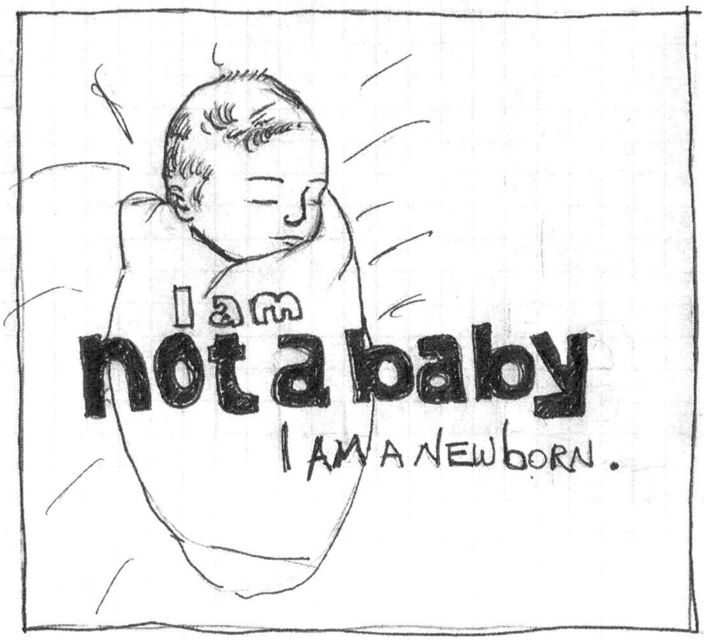

Fig. 6.1 "I am not a baby" branding campaign for Enfamil, a baby formula. Printed matter and free samples of Enfamil were mailed to me during my miscarriage. Illustration by the author, 2016.

a newborn." This envelope has taken on the significance of a magical, powerful object for this detective (Layne 2000a, p. 132; Mitchell 2005, pp. 121–24). This is not an envelope, no, it is an object that is transubstantiated through the algorithmic and branding powers of direct marketing, and activated—enlivened—with significance, symbolism, affect, and kinship. It is a fetish (Marx 1976, vol. 1, pp. 163–65). Through the power of big data marketing analytics, this envelope becomes a commodity fetish, enlivened and crackling with the social relations that went into its making. I was dispossessed of my health data through the network of health data disclosure, only for it to come back to me in the form of this targeted, personalized marketing.

You might assume that I "own" this envelope, as it was mailed directly to me and since the day that it was delivered, has been in my exclusive possession. Yet, when I contacted Mead Johnson Inc., the manufacturers of Enfamil, for permission to reprint an image of it in this book, they turned down my request, especially after I refused their counter-request that I send them the chapter I was writing about the advertisement for their approval. This denial of reprint permission underlined for me again that despite the fact that I possess a material representation of my health data, (in this case a piece of direct marketing mail), the object is not mine, just as my data is not mine. It is owned by a company: Mead Johnson in the case of the envelope, Experian in the case of my data, and any number of direct marketers that own my "consumer data profile." Michael Taussig, an economic anthropologist who writes about commodities, fetishes, and power that both possess says that the power of drawings, as opposed to photographs, is in their ability to encompass time. Drawings, unlike photographs or even words, "intervene in the reckoning of reality" (Taussig 2011, p. 13). If a photograph is taken to be a depiction of "what is real," then a drawing disrupts the notion that reality can be captured and translated verbatim by a technological device (Mitchell 2005). Of course, this is a fallacy, as photographs create their own reality, just as much as drawings do. The reality that I am capturing through my hand-drawn illustration of a piece of evidence from my marketing baby's body is one of ownership, of affect, of kinship. If I cannot own the photograph of my marketing baby or even the data that went in to its birth, then I will *draw* it to *own* it. I will draw my desires for kinship ties, my affections, my love, though thwarted, so that these might live again in ink and paper. This piece of printed, folded paper, as well as my drawing of it, to paraphrase both Karen Barad and W.J.T. Mitchell, is matter that *matters*. It shows that my ephemeral data revenant has a body, it has a voice, and it demands to be heard (Mitchell 2005, p. 153; Barad 2003). Through my drawing of the evidence of my marketing baby's body, too, I take back some control over my data image from marketers who claim to own it.

The Immaterial Gets "Real"

What is this thing, my marketing baby? Is it the ghostly image of my data, interpreted by marketers as a living, breathing baby? Is it a golem condemned to roam the data warehouses of the American desert? Is it a data changeling, activated by marketing trolls and fairies to do their bidding? Is it a flat data image, or a representation that is so life-like it is uncanny? Flat but made fleshy and enlivened through its transformation into a data commodity that takes on a life of its own (Marx 1976, vol. 1, p. 128)? Am I to be blamed for my own haunting, like Ester blamed herself for her data revenant in Chapter 1? Did I make this creature not out of mud and charnel-house materials, but out of my personal information that I carelessly released into the world, through my loyalty card swipes, through my Google searches, through my signing away of my digital privacy (Shelley 2003)?[5]

What are we to make of my data baby, embodied as it is in this bit of marketing material? For the entirety of this noir, dear reader, this humble detective pursued a mysterious person, and now finds herself confronted with the object of her investigation. One of the most striking things about my marketing baby's flat fleshiness is that it echoes René Magritte's 1929 painting *The Treachery of Images.* The painting has become a canonical example of surrealism and of the instability between language, images, and the material world. The painting contains an image of a pipe, rendered somewhat "realistically," floating in a neutral field of beige oil paint. Painted underneath, in a cursive script, is the emphatic phrase "*Ceci n'est pas une pipe*" [this is not a pipe]. Through the image and text, Magritte presents us with a riddle. The painting itself is an object, and it is also an image depicting an object. It is also a sign, a material, conceptual, and emotional thing with a linguistic signification, a sign that is also depicted as an image in the word "pipe." Magritte's painting embodies the perpetual tension and instability between the subject and the thing, between the immaterial and the material, between the concept and the object. In her book *The Wretched of the Screen*, Hito Steyerl argues for the life-like fullness and plumpness of digital images (2013). Of the digital image's agency she writes, "[s]enses and things, abstraction and excitement, speculation and power, desire and matter actually converge within images. … [t]his image is not some ideological misconception, but a thing simultaneously couched in affect and availability, a fetish made of crystals and electricity, animated by our wishes and fears—a perfect embodiment of its own conditions of existence. … The bruises of things are deciphered, and then subjected to interpretation. Things are made to speak—often by subjecting them to additional violence" (Steyerl 2013, p. 52).

This envelope poses a similar riddle to me as Magritte's painting. The envelope is simultaneously an object, an image, and the material and symbolic manifestation of my lack of a living child. "I am not a baby." No you're not … but you are. The object, the thing, the data commodity speaks (Arvatov and Kiaer 1997, p. 126). It says that it is not what it appears to be, but I can see exactly what it is. I made this baby through my body, through my desires, and through my health traumas, but instead of being made of my genetic material, this baby was made of my health and consumer data.[6]

Perhaps I can trace my marketing baby, born of dead matter and digital information, to middle-class Victorians who would have photographic portraits made of their dead children, seated or standing in "life-like" poses or positioned among their living siblings and parents (Blood and Cacciatore 2014).[7] Media scholars Michele White and Lisa Nakamura, along with sociologist Linda Layne theorize how a miscarried fetus' immateriality is articulated via digital media and made "real," touchable, and "life-like" (White 2010, 2015; Nakamura 2008; Layne 2000a, b). One of the ways the immateriality of trauma is made in flesh is in the phenomenon of the Reborn dolls that White writes about. Reborn dolls are manufactured vinyl dolls that are recrafted by enthusiasts, who customize off-the-shelf dolls' heads, torsos and limbs into very realistic looking figures of newly born babies. White carefully, and often tenderly, analyzes the women artists and "mothers" who create the uncanny Reborn baby dolls, some of which are made to memorialize their miscarried, stillborn, or dead children. Such dolls are available for "adoption" on eBay and other auction sites, thus given a life beyond death. While this form of life may look like a substitute for the real one that never was, for those mothers who give birth to Reborn dolls, the "babies" are alive with their affect. Both Nakamura's analysis of emoticons and other digital ephemera created by women who have miscarried or had stillborn babies and Layne's analysis of ways that women memorialize their miscarried babies using ultrasound images demonstrate how immaterial things, or at least things that are inaccessible to one's touch or gaze, are rematerialized. They are given an ersatz life to participate in affective and kinship networks: Dead things are reborn online, through images and data. All of these are commodity fetishes in the sense that they are the material (and immaterial) manifestation of social relations. They are objects that are animated with affective relations; they are not merely pixels on a screen or finely painted plastic. Their value inheres in the emotional response that they evoke in those who create and possess them. Although Michael Taussig describes commodity fetishes as denoting "an attribution of life, autonomy, power, and even dominance to otherwise inanimate objects and presupposes a draining of these qualities from the human actors who bestow the attribution" to things, I, along with these grieving mothers, am twisting the power of the fetish back on itself (Taussig 2010, pp. 31–32).

For me, my marketing baby is more than a collection of infant formula canisters or printed brochures that promote child life insurance. I drain the agential force of these marketing artifacts, objects sent to me in a bid to persuade me to buy goods and participate in the grand capitalist masquerade that hides its injustices in the shiny objects it produces. No, instead of letting the fetish drain me, I take these bits of paper and powdered milk, mix in my tears and the bloody detritus of my womb, and fill this dead thing with a new life free of the branded mothering of Gerber or Met Life, and full of my own tenderness, my own anger, and my own desires. I fill my marketing baby with my own meaning.

Boris Arvatov, a Russian Constructivist art critic and historian, proposed that the ultimate revolutionary act is to make commodities intimate, especially commodities alienated from those who produce them, to make them kin (Arvatov and Kiaer 1997). Arvatov's 1925 essay "Everyday Life and the Culture of the Thing (Toward the Formulation of the Question)," is almost prescient in its description of the ways that we attach emotional and affective meanings to consumer commodities, things, and thus, the power of things is unleashed through our relationships to them and through them. Arvatov asks us to reimagine a thing, an object, that is "*differently* animated from the commodity fetish … [and by doing so] there is an attempt to return a kind of social agency to the fetish" (Kiaer 1997, p. 111, emphasis in the original). Objects, like my marketing baby, can be inserted into my affective kinship networks, and made to perform social work that my miscarriage could not. A colleague of Arvatov's, Alexander Rodchenko, argued for the liberation of things, along with people, from the status of mere commodity. Through this release from the enslavement of consumption, we should see things integrated into our social worlds as friends, comrades, and lovers: "Objects will be understood, will become people's friends and comrades, and people will begin to know how to laugh and enjoy and converse with things" (quoted in Kravets 2013, p. 421).

This is how I see my marketing baby. Through freeing it from the conditions and the intentions of its "birth" in Experian's Marketing Services databases, I take it into my arms, hold it, and call this marketing baby my own flesh and blood. It turns out, as in most noirs, the mysterious person I've been searching for is both my baby, constructed by database marketing, and myself. I am the commodity as well. The subject becomes an object. A fleshy, lively being becomes a thing. A thing is born out of dead matter.

Notes

1. Dr. Bruno Ludenfeld, the inventor of manufactured FSH, was interviewed in 2011 about this history. He said, "it turned out that the Vatican owned a majority of the shares in the Serono company. So, with a direct request from the Pope's nephew, Don Giulio Pacelli, who was a member of the Serono Board of Directors, it was easy to get the cooperation of nuns living in old-age homes throughout Italy" (Dichek 2011). The brand name GONAL-F is now owned by EMD Serono Inc., a division of Merck Inc.
2. The direct-to-consumer website of the drug PREMARIN® is found at https://www.premarin.com.
3. Preciado places himself within this matrix in *Testo Junkie*, Chap. 8.
4. Schering-Plough was purchased by Merck Inc. in 2009 in a $41.1-billion merger. The Schering-Plough Research Institute was still operational and conducting drug investigations in 2011 during the PURSUE study. In 2013, the FDA accepted Merck Inc.'s New Drug Application for standard review of the PURSUE study drug, corifollitropin alfa (Eisele 2013).
5. Perhaps I also shared Victor Frankenstein's hubris when he similarly threw together the materials of life to make his Creature, thinking that all that is needed to make life out of nothing is a passionate intelligence and material resources.
6. As of August 2015, Experian Marketing Services Inc. had 34 patent applications for various algorithms, database structures, and data processes, and 33 issued patents. Information on US patent holders is found at http://www.uspto.gov.
7. The practice of memorializing stillbirths in family photographs continues in the twenty-first century. The website www.nowilaymedowntosleep.org provides volunteer photographers who will come to the hospital rooms of grieving parents to create loving portraits of stillborn and premature babies.

References

Althusser, Louis. 2001. *Lenin and Philosophy and Other Essays*. Translated by Ben Brewster. New York: Monthly Review Press.

Arvatov, Boris, and Christina Kiaer. 1997. "Everyday Life and the Culture of the Thing (Toward the Formulation of the Question)." *October* 81 (2): 119–28.

Barad, Karen. 2003. "Posthumanist Performativity: Toward an Understanding of How Matter Comes to Matter." *Signs* 28 (3): 801–31.

Blood, Cybele, and Joanne Cacciatore. 2014. "Parental Grief and Memento Mori Photography: Narrative, Meaning, Culture, and Context." *Death Studies* 38 (4): 224–33.

Brown, Bill. 2001. "Thing Theory." *Critical Inquiry* 28 (1): 1–22.

Chamberlain, Simon, Harley Giles, and Andrew Lientz. 2015. "Service for Associating Network Users with Profiles." United States Patent and Trademark Office 9,058,340, filed September 9, 2013, and issued June 16, 2015.

Cheney-Lippold, John. 2011. "A New Algorithmic Identity: Soft Biopolitics and the Modulation of Control." *Theory, Culture & Society* 28 (6): 164–81.

Dichek, Bernard. 2011. "Baby Boomer." *Israel21c: Uncovering Israel*, February 8. Accessed January 9, 2016. http://www.israel21c.org/baby-boomer.

Eisele, Pam. 2013. "Merck Announces FDA Acceptance of New Drug Application for Investigational Fertility Treatment." Press Release. Whitehouse Station, NJ: Merck. http://www.drugs.com/nda/corifollitropin_alfa_130909.html.

Engel, William E., and Max F. Kigler. 2013. "Process and System for Integrating Information from Disparate Databases for Purposes of Predicting Consumer Behavior." United States Patent and Trademark Office 8,612,282, filed May 3, 2012, and issued December 17, 2013.

Freud, Sigmund. 2003. *The Uncanny*. Translated by David Mclintock. London: Penguin Classics.

Haraway, Donna. 1997. *Modest_Witness@Second_Millennium.FemaleMan©_Meets_OncoMouse™: Feminism and Technoscience*. New York: Routledge.

———. 2008. *When Species Meet*. Minneapolis: University of Minnesota Press.

Kiaer, Christina. 1997. "Boris Arvatov's Socialist Objects." *October* 81 (2): 105–18.

Kravets, Olga. 2013. "On Things and Comrades." *Ephemera* 13 (2): 421–36.

Layne, Linda L. 2000a. "Baby Things as Fetishes: Memorial Goods, Simulacra, and the 'Realness' Problem of Pregnancy Loss." In *Ideologies and Technologies of Motherhood: Race, Class, Sexuality, Nationalism*, edited by Heléna Ragoné and France Winddance Twine, 111–38. New York: Routledge.

———. 2000b. "'He Was a Real Baby with Baby Things': A Material Culture Analysis of Personhood, Parenthood and Pregnancy Loss." *Journal of Material Culture* 5 (3): 321–45.

Markham, Annette N. 2013. "The Algorithmic Self: Layered Accounts of Life and Identity in the 21st Century." *Selected Papers of Internet Research* 14: 1–4.

Marx, Karl. 1976. *Capital: A Critique of Political Economy*. Vol. 1. Translated by Ben Fowkes. London: Penguin.

Mitchell, W. J. T. 2005. *What Do Pictures Want? The Lives and Loves of Images*. Chicago: University of Chicago Press.

Nakamura, Lisa. 2008. *Digitizing Race: Visual Cultures of the Internet*. Minneapolis: University of Minnesota Press.

Preciado, Paul B. 2013. *Testo Junkie: Sex, Drugs, and Biopolitics in the Pharmacopornographic Era*. Kindle. New York: Feminist Press.

Rajan, Kaushik Sunder. 2006. *Biocapital: The Constitution of Postgenomic Life*. Durham, NC: Duke University Press.

Robertson, Jordan, and Shannon Pettypiece. 2014. "They Know You Buy Viagra and They Want to Sell You More." *Bloomberg Business*, December 10. Accessed January 9, 2016. http://www.bloomberg.com/news/articles/2014-12-10/they-know-you-buy-viagra-and-they-want-to-sell-you-more.

Rose, Nikolas. 2007. *The Politics of Life Itself: Biomedicine, Power, and Subjectivity in the Twenty-First Century*. Princeton, NJ: Princeton University Press.

Shelley, Mary. 2003. *Frankenstein: Or the Modern Prometheus*. London: Penguin Classics.

Solove, Daniel J. 2006. *The Digital Person: Technology and Privacy in the Information Age*. New York: New York University Press.

Steyerl, Hito. 2013. *The Wretched of the Screen*. New York: Sternberg Press.

Taussig, Michael. 2010. *Devil and Commodity Fetishism in South America*. 2nd ed. Chapel Hill: University of North Carolina Press.

———. 2011. *I Swear I Saw This: Drawings in Fieldwork Notebooks, Namely Mine*. Chicago: University of Chicago Press.

Thompson, Charis. 1999. "Confessions of a Bioterrorist: Subject Position and Reproductive Technologies." In *Playing Dolly: Technocultural Formations, Fantasies and Fictions in Assisted Reproduction*, edited by E. Ann Kaplan and Susan Squier, 189–240. New Brunswick, NJ: Rutgers University Press.

Timmermans, Stefan. 2010. "Reconciling Research with Medical Care in RCTs." In *Medical Proofs, Social Experiments: Clinical Trials in Shifting Contexts*, edited by Catherine Will and Tiago Moreira, 17–32. Farnham, UK: Ashgate.

Waldby, Catherine, and Melinda Cooper. 2010. "From Reproductive Work to Regenerative Labour: The Female Body and the Stem Cell Industries." *Feminist Theory* 11 (1): 3–22.

Waldby, Catherine, and Robert Mitchell. 2006. *Tissue Economies: Blood, Organs, and Cell Lines in Late Capitalism*. Durham, NC: Duke University Press.

White, Michele. 2010. "Babies Who Touch You: Reborn Dolls, Artists, and the Emotive Display of Bodies on eBay." In *Political Emotions*, edited by Janet Staiger, Ann Cvetkovich, and Ann Reynolds, 66–89. London: Routledge.

———. 2015. *Producing Women: The Internet, Traditional Femininity, Queerness, and Creativity*. London: Routledge.

CHAPTER 7

The Body of Evidence

My marketing baby's bones and flesh of direct mail marketing and customized online ads have become the body of evidence for my hard-boiled investigation; that pile of bones speaks to me and taunts me to pursue it, to find it, to make it whole again. This body of evidence has my name on it (see Fig. 7.1). It gurgles and coos: "go to South Boston."

Southie is what the residents of this historically working-class—and now gentrifying—neighborhood call it. A community of long-time and newer residents, who live side-by-side in redeveloped waterfront properties, warehouses-cum-luxury condos, or nineteenth-century row houses and older public housing blocks. Some houses appear to be long vacated by poorer residents, while others remain in homes passed down through generations. Freshly painted and well-appointed cheese shops with names like *Fromage* and gastro pubs called *The Lincoln* incongruously abut the shabbiness of the discount dollar stores, the South Boston community health center, and corners festooned with Irish flags. Southie boasts some of the most expensive real estate in Boston, which contrast sharply with the neighborhood's historic home prices. It was not that long ago that these streets were controlled, and terrorized, by mob boss James "Whitey" Bulger, and signs of community struggles still visibly mark the neighborhood. The day I arrived was unseasonably cold and blustery. As I walked north on Dorchester Street toward the bay, I turned up my collar to keep the wind off my neck. I caught something out of the corner of my eye: a flyer taped to a shop window announcing a public vigil for those who have

M.F.E. Ebeling, *Healthcare and Big Data*,
DOI 10.1057/978-1-137-50221-6_7

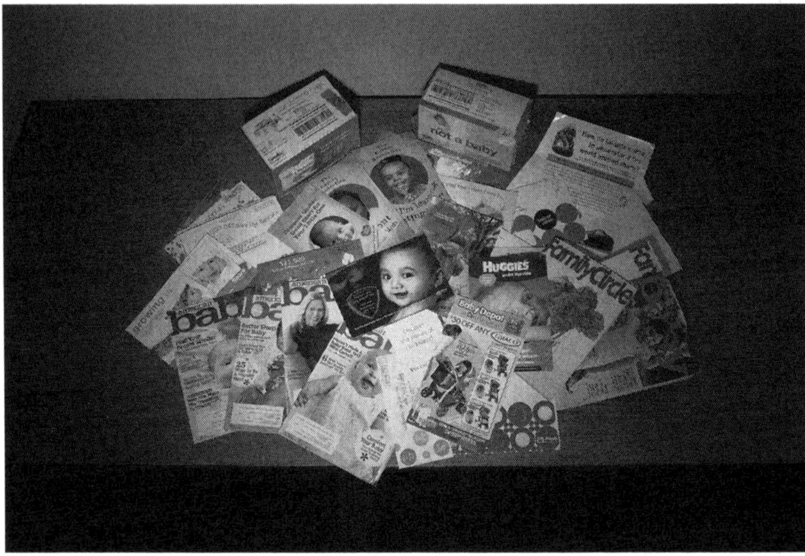

Fig. 7.1 The Body of Evidence. Credit: Jay Muhlin 2016.

died from drug overdoses. The hardscrabble live cheek-to-jowl with the well-heeled in these parts.

I wondered aloud, speaking only to myself, how the data analysts working on Experian's Mosaic market segmentation tool would categorize the residents of this neighborhood. Certainly they would plunk the neighborhood into "Urban Essence," "Aspiring Contemporatires [*sic*]," or "Struggling Societies" but then what (Experian Marketing Services 2009, p. 2)? How to subcategorize the diversity of struggles and aspirations that no doubt these residents experienced every day? "Metro Beginnings?" "Struggling City Centers?" "Minority Metro Communities?" "Getting By?" The essence of people's private traumas boiled down, dried, and sliced up to be sold.

"So, I'm supposed to find my marketing baby here, in Southie?" I mumbled to myself as I walked toward my destination: the Direct Marketing Association's (DMA) annual conference "&Then."

I arrived at the Boston Convention and Exhibition Center, a hulking mass of concrete and glass that faced east toward the bay, and entered into one of the largest trade shows for the data marketing industry in the USA, possibly the world. I had been told by several sources that if there was any place that I was going to find my marketing baby, it would be the DMA.

During the entirety of my sleuthing work, I had not had the opportunity to meet my marketing baby's midwives—the data analysts, data engineers, and data brokers who collated, chopped up, and reassembled my data into sellable data assets—but now they would all be in one place. In fact, Experian Marketing Services, the one data broker that Eliza named as a confirmed source that had sold my data, was scheduled to be on the convention floor. At that point, the company had responded with frustrating silence to my several requests to speak to a person at Experian or to obtain a full copy of all of the data and data sources that Experian holds on me to put together my data image. I even went as far as to recruit a data rights watchdog organization, Request Initiative, and through the group's lawyer, Samir Dathi,[1] had sent Experian a data subject request. Experian responded by sending me an unsolicited copy of my credit report. After this failed attempt to receive my data, I found buried on the Experian website a way of requesting my marketing data from the company—I had to print off a request form, along with a photocopy of my driver's license, as well as two copies of utility bills addressed to me, and mail it to a PO box in Texas. Six weeks later, I received a brief, "consumer marketing report" which contained bare-bone and generalized information on me, not the information that I requested. I decided to treat the DMA convention as the site of the final "showdown" with Experian.[2] I suspected that some of my data that Experian captured came from the credit card transactions that I made in the fertility clinic—$25,000 worth. I was determined to find someone at the trade show who could confirm that my detective hunches were right: My marketing baby was built, at least in part, from transactional data.

My investigations into the information circuits that are covered under HIPAA and through which my data traversed led me to more questions than answers, and only deepened my confusion and uncertainty about where I might find my baby. I began my detective work fiercely determined to master the network of disclosure, to understand the complex, totality of the system, to hunt down the company that owned my baby, and to have a final confrontation. I fantasized a lot about how the final confrontation would go down: I would march through the door of their low-slung, prefab, business-park building and demand to hold my baby, to feel the weight and warmth of its data body in my arms, look down and coo into its pixel eyes.

Despite this imagined triumph, I found myself ensnared once again in a trap electrified by futile desires, as I was similarly entangled for four years in the fertility industry's hormonally amplified web of aspirational fecundity. And I was about to enter the lair of aspirational consumerism. The pursuits of both my fleshly and my digital baby were propelled and sustained by false hopes. Thus fueled and sustained, I followed some of the leads and clues that I had scribbled down in my detective's notebook during my interviews with informants.

In Boston that day, I was hopeful that after years of glimpses and senses (but never full head-on looks), finally I could come face-to-face with my baby made of data. The final challenge was nigh. The banners that streamed from the vaulted steel beam ceilings advertised the data analytics companies that were present in the trade show. One particularly caught my eye, for the Belgium-based company Selligent. The banner featured a photograph of a European male, who appeared affluent (perhaps it was the haircut, the freshly-scrubbed fair skin, the collar of a tailor-made shirt peeking out from under an expensive jacket, the positioning of the model in a first-class lounge, the serene expression?), softly smiling as he looked at his smart phone. The banner's text read: "Enhance the Moment" and "John, your flight is now boarding." The banner emblematizes what the direct marketing industry is striving for: personalized marketing to identifiable individuals. The Selligent marketing services representatives that I spoke to at the convention used phrases like "moment of engagement," "delivering personalized brand experiences," and "hyperconnection" to describe their offerings. Unlike health informatics or financial analytics researchers, who use large, aggregated, and anonymized datasets (say data derived from census tracts) to study overall trends or the movement of a social or economic phenomenon, data marketers use big data to narrow in on individual "prospects" and target identifiable consumers with marketing. Of course, data marketers also conduct analyses to identify trends, but in the case of targeted marketing, the aim is to drill down to an identifiable person. In the promotional text for one of Experian Marketing Services' analytical tools, for example, a tool to help marketers identify a single costumer, notes that "[u]nderstanding your customer's identity and behavior across channels is crucial to developing and sharing your brand story effectively" (Experian Marketing Services 2016). In "From Big Data to Big Marketing," a white paper by Fair Isaac Corporation (FICO), the developers of the FICO score, a graphic explains how big data analytics can tunnel through mass sets of data to single out an individual, identifiable consumer, in this case pictured as a young, smiling, white woman holding four colorful shopping bags, her image under a magnifying glass (Fair Isaac Corporation 2012, p. 3).

Direct marketing has its origins in developing mailing lists based on data from the US Postal Service and the White Pages (R.R. Donnelly, the publisher of phone directories was at the &Then conference in Boston, as was the US Postal Service) to send direct mailings of promotional materials to customers. In the era of big data, social media, and online marketing, what was once applied to paper records, marketers now apply sophisticated algorithms to massive databases to identify and profile a single person. As I described in Chapter 2, segmentation marketing is the process by which data on virtually every US household are divvied up into marketing categories. Target marketing uses these segmented data to tailor messages to the customers that are most likely to read the email or the mailer on top of all the junk mail. Target marketing endeavors to cut through the continuous stream of marketing messages (US consumers are exposed to about 5,000 marketing message *per day*), and capture the attention of the prospects most likely to be converted into long-term customers.

Data Paranoia

Some of us respond with "data paranoia" to the uncanny ability of target marketers, who use browser tools and other algorithmic "magic" to predict what we are thinking and what we desire before we even know it. This grows out of our worries about how our data, especially data that we produce from our online behaviors, is being tracked by forces that we know exist but remain nameless and faceless, a big "They."

About a year ago, Toshi, a filmmaker who used to produce advertising campaigns for pharmaceutical companies, noticed a curious phenomenon. During an interview about how her health information was coming back to haunt her online, she told me a story that illustrated for her "data paranoia." When she searched for a product that she needed, in the example she offered, a consumer-end laser printer for her home office, she began receiving emails from Amazon.com offering her the same item she was searching for. Knowing not to fall for Amazon's "click bait" by clicking through the link to the sale item, she deleted the first email. A week later, she received another unsolicited email from Amazon, which said: "We noticed you didn't purchase the printer, it is still on sale." She said of the experience:

> It has been bothering me. At first I thought it was creepy, but now I think this is the new paradigm that we live with, and now I've come to accept it, and it's not right to accept this. Why is it that I accept it? I feel there is an

> informational overload and I can't keep track. When I see these things pop in [emails and pop-up advertisements] all within the past year, I see this as the new norm, and it doesn't have that sting any more, and it should.

When faced with the fact that this type of data surveillance by target marketers is the new norm, at first we may be appalled. But then many of us learn to accept it, and even to ignore it. Target marketers are aware of this, and innovate new ways to target customers knowing that we will delete and ignore their messages. Toshi's example illustrates target marketing quite well, as data-based direct marketing's goal is to have total data surveillance across all media platforms so that marketers can send relevant and highly targeted communications directly to individuals. It does not matter, for the databases, whether one is looking for a printer or for information about diabetes; all of this data will be swept up and spat back out to us in the form of direct marketing. Target marketers want to follow us across all of the media platforms that we use—our phones, computers, Internet-connected televisions, junk mail—to engage us in personalized and intimate conversations about the stuff we buy.

At the conference in Boston, I found my way through the maze of exhibitor booths filled with tat—squeeze balls, plush toys, pens, key chains, USB thumb drives, mini-speakers, magnets, Moscow Mule copper mugs (filled with the iced vodka cocktail), shopping bags—all emblazoned with a company's logo and placed on tables to entice conventioneers to take a longer look. There was even a whole section of the convention floor featuring vendors who market promotional products. I came across the Selligent booth, the Belgian data marketing firm introduced earlier. I couldn't resist the Belgian waffles and cappuccinos they were offering, so I stopped and listened while munching. I learned that Selligent is a customer relationship management (CRM) platform company, providing software that helps companies interact with their customers through websites, online retail transactions, emails, and mobile communications. CRM firms may also provide data analytic support on the data that is collected through their platform by the licensees who purchase the software. These companies are similar to the credit bureaus and electronic health records vendors that also provide software that collects customer data in order to perform data analytics.

In addition to the companies working in data acquisition, data compilation, data hygiene, list compilation, and mailing and printing services, Experian was present on the trade show floor. Experian's representation, however, was limited to their marketing and data hygiene services. Data hygiene refers to "cleaning up" data for sale. In Chapter 4, I described how retail and specialty pharmacies sell de-identified prescription information to data brokers, such as IMS Health Inc.: Patient's identifiers are replaced with numerical codes as a way to de-identify patients' protected health information and be compliant with HIPAA regulations. And in the network of disclosure, there are third-party companies that specialize in data security to de-identify records. Similarly, there are also third-party companies that conduct "data hygiene": submitting datasets to algorithms specifically programmed to clean up data. What characterizes "clean data" for the data marketing industry? Clean data is *accurate* information (as much as is possible, given technical and regulatory constraints) about a person's name, mailing address, number of children in the household, income level, inferred or self-reported race, ethnicity and gender, home ownership, political affinities, and inferred "interests" (ranging from diseases or health conditions to sports and hobbies).[3] Data hygienists aim to produce data commodities that are finely grained, highly reliable, and precise, to sell to direct marketers.

At the DMA conference, I heard and saw several mantras repeated, including "We Live Data," "We Make Connections," "Individualized Insights," "Engage Your Customers through the Omnichannel Journey," and "Connect. Cultivate. Convert."[4] Some of the more intriguing claims about what these data management companies can do caught my attention: company claims to delve into a customer's "DNA," advertisements proclaiming that the digital revolution means a marketing evolution, the words "Adapt or Die" overlaid on an image of Charles Darwin. In fact, I have seen this connection made between marketing data and genetics quite a few times outside the trade show as well, in places like marketing white papers, downloaded from the websites of Experian Marketing Services and McKinsey Digital (the data marketing arm of the consulting firm McKinsey & Co.), with titles such as "Mapping Your Customer's DNA: A CMO Imperative" (Experian Marketing Services 2015) or "Cracking the Digital-Shopper Genome" (BenMark and Maher 2015). It seems that the data marketing industry has borrowed the genetic code and evolutionary metaphors of post-humanist media scholars such as Eugene Thacker or N. Katherine Hayles to describe the embodiment of consumption and how, through the use of data analytics, a marketer can perform a "vivisection" upon a customer's digital body to make her "reveal her (shopping) secrets" (Hayles 1999; Thacker 2003a, b; Merchant 2008). Thacker, who looks at how biologists use computational DNA, and Hayles, who studies cybernetic information, both lay bare "the cultural perception that information and materiality are conceptually distinct and that information is in some sense more essential, more important and more fundamental than materiality" (Hayles 1999, p. 18). Materiality instantiates data, and although data marketers use a different language, they too mine (and profit from) the materiality of data.

In my wanderings around the convention floor, I came upon a vendor's booth that I thought might be able to help me understand what happens to credit and debit card transactional data. In its promotional materials, the company described itself as providing "strategic solutions for insurance and financial services companies looking to advance and improve their direct marketing strategy" (Direct Marketing Association 2015). At the booth, I found Arun Nichani, a financial data expert who worked out of the company's New York City office, and a self-described "data geek." Perhaps he could help me understand what happens to the transactional data that results from making card payments at a clinic or hospital.

Nichani was friendly and excited to share with me what he knew about transactional data. He explained how these data move out of a doctor's office when a credit card is swiped: When you hand over your card for a co-payment or for a self-pay procedure transaction, the doctor's office swipes your card using a point-of-sale terminal, sometimes called a "rail," that collects key information from both the transaction and from the patient's card. This information is transferred to the card processing company, using the hardwired terminal the processing company set up in the doctor's office. In the USA, the two dominant card processors are First Credit and Chase Paymentech. The card is swiped and the data is broken up into three levels: The first level contains data for transactions made between a consumer and a business using a consumer credit or debit card; the second level is for business-to-business transactions using a corporate-issued card; and the third level is for corporate- or government-issued cards and transactions (Jennings 2015).

Level one data has the fewest details about the transaction. It includes the doctor's merchant category code, the unique identifying code for each terminal (which will also include the name of the doctor's office and the location), the amount of the transaction, and the date of the transaction. Nichani used the example of the level-one transactional data generated when I used my VISA credit card, a card issued through my bank, J.P. Morgan Chase—the *issuing bank* is Chase and Visa is the *network* or the "brand" of the card. Nichani explained what transactional data at level one typically will look like to the issuing bank and to the network:

> Nichani: [Chase will] know that it's $25 and there will be that MCC code that gets assigned, which is the merchant category code. This classification is very important because this allows Chase to identify that do you qualify for the 5 percent bonus this quarter. They use that; they're doing some analytics on this. They want to know what sort of expenses was [*sic*]. They'll probably know that it's a healthcare related [transaction], patients probably they will certainly know it's healthcare related. That's the extent of information they have.
>
> Mary: Will they have my doctor's name?
>
> Nichani: Oh yes. If it's a practice with 10 doctors, they won't have every doctor's name, but they'll have all the details. They know exactly where this card was swiped. They know exactly who that business belongs to. First Data[5] assuming, or in this case it would be Chase Paymentech who sold the terminal to the doctor. Chase Paymentech has all of that information in one system. Are they all talking to each other? Maybe not yet, but eventually that's the goal that all the issuers, all the networks want to do is how to do more analytics with this information. They're starting to, in some cases, resell this information.

That information, that issuers and networks are reselling transactional data, perked up my ears. I verified what Nichani told me against a shareholders' seminar report I found on Experian's "investor relations" website detailing Experian's purchase of data on one billion consumer MasterCard transactions, as well a *Wall Street Journal* article detailing the technology that data brokers and card networks use to link credit card transactional data made in offline retailers to online ads served to a cardholder, much like the prescription matchbacks described in Chapter 6 (Steel 2011; Robert 2013, p. 8). In fact, VISA holds a patent for an algorithm that could potentially be used to link a cardholder's DNA to their consumer profile (Steel 2011). These types of data sales are the "business-as-usual" transactions of data marketers.

Nichani went on to explain that certain card networks, namely Discover Card and American Express, are both the processor and the network. This way, they have more control over the data that moves through the transactional network, and it is easier for them to submit the data to valuable analytics, because they hold the data and do not have to collate the data from other owners. Retailers hold transactional data that is very valuable to issuing banks and card networks because the retailers have a record of the items purchased during a transaction. There are new companies that have entered the field to address a gap in data access: e-commerce transaction companies. For example, Slice, an online consumer platform that enables users to organize and keep track of their online and offline purchases through e-receipts and emails, has figured out how to get at transactional data directly through the cardholder. The platform follows the social media model and, just like Facebook, Slice offers the tool for "free" to users—cardholders—in exchange for access to their very valuable data. Slice then owns all of the transactional data within a customer's receipt, so that even if a purchase was made through Target.com and Target claims proprietary ownership of the transactional data, Slice can do an end run around it by scraping the data from the customer's use of the Slice platform. Slice can then sell or lease that information to another party for analytics, marketing, or other uses.

Experian Owns Us

Nichani also explained to me that holders of consumer credit data are always looking for new ways to innovate upon it. As mentioned in Chapter 2, many data services companies use disparate sources of information to innovate new products and assets. Some of these innovations include the use of data that seems unrelated, such as posts that a user may make to Facebook or social media, to be combined with another source of data, such as a person's Fair Isaac Corporation (FICO) credit risk score, to construct a "three-dimensional" data image of an individual. While on the face of it, it may seem that this is a business-as-usual operation for data brokers, for certain kinds of data, such as those that are related to finance or health, this can have serious implications. It's these sorts of innovations that Nichani found worrisome, in particular how credit bureaus are seeking to incorporate customers' social media use, health risk factors, and ethnicity in credit risk scores. He described these developments as a type of "data red-lining." It is through this type of data red-lining that companies such as Experian own us, not only do they own our data but they potentially own our life chances as well, through the determination of our credit risk based on data that may or may not have anything to do with our creditworthiness but has more to do with "social engineering." Another concern about these innovations is the ability of card issuers or networks to combine transactional data with a card user's phone to provide real time advertisements:

> [T]hey're calling it geo-fencing. What that is, is the second you swipe that card at your doctor's office, all the businesses in the vicinity [near the doctor's office] and based on, [where] they know [a card holder is at the time of the transaction in real time] ... Let's say you shop at the Gap. If they know that you are likely to shop at the Gap, they'll send you an offer at that time for a discount or a deal or some percentage [discount] at Gap as soon as you swipe there. Because they know that the Gap store is less than 500 feet from your doctor's office. ... [So] you're in your doctor's office, you swipe [your card] ... As soon as you swipe, now VISA and Chase know where you are, because they know the physical location of the terminal that the card was swiped at [and can send you advertisements for the Gap that may be next door to your doctor's office]. Once they know, and that's why they call it ... geographical fencing. Now they hone in and they zone in and they go, 'Ah. this is where she's at.' Is there any other business around here that we want [to target her for because she frequents it] ... and they want to touch you [with personalized and targeted advertising] when it's relevant. Because you'll tune them out very quick if they are unnecessarily bothering you. That's the game that they have to play smart."

While we were talking, I built up my courage, sensing that I may have found an ally, another comrade. I told Nichani that I was actually not a sociologist, but a detective in the middle of a case. I told him about my marketing baby. Nichani was astonished: "how could this happen? This I could say I think it's wrong." He speculated about some of the ways that that my marketing baby could have been born, and for him it came down to algorithmic identities:

> [N]ow they're able to infer that if this is the case that's happening right here. That's probably what it is. It's all these disjointed sets, which historically could never have been connected but today they are. ... Because this is not [a] human [putting it together], this is all algorithms at work.

Before I left Nichani's exhibition booth, he offered me an idea about how I might finally get all of my data from Experian. He asked me, "Have you filed a complaint with the Consumer Financial Protection Bureau?" I told him I had not, that I hadn't even thought it was possible to do so. I thought that the Consumer Financial Protection Bureau (CFPB), a governmental agency originally proposed by economist and consumer credit rights advocate Senator Elizabeth Warren (D-MA) and founded under the Obama Administration, was a consumer financial rights watchdog and regulator that only handled complaints against banks, not against credit bureaus and data marketing companies (Eichelberger 2014). I promised him that I would look into it. With that bit of advice, as I suspected, Nichani was indeed a comrade.

Empathy and the Violence of "Dumb" Data

As I mentioned in previous chapters, bureaucracies, databases and data contain within them the potency of structural violence, which if triggered, can be unleashed to produce material harm. As media scholar Daniel Solove, who has written a lot about databases, summarized quite neatly the trauma my marketing baby has caused me as well as how the data industry, while they may not intend to, inadvertently, do cause harm as discussed in Chapter 6 (Solove 2006a, b). Often times, this harm is wrought by "dumb" data, or data that is inaccurate (and in a certain sense all data owned by data brokers is dumb) or that inadequately reflects the complexities of our lives. Data's violence is in its flattening of its subjects—us—into a data image that can never capture the full dimensionality of our vitality, no matter how sophisticated a marketer's algorithm may be.

During my fieldwork at the convention, I asked virtually every data broker and analyst that agreed to speak with me if they could help me find my marketing baby. Could they help me reassemble its data body—how was it conceived, where it was born, where does it live now, how old is it? Is it lonely, does it miss me when it is dispersed across databases or within the data warehouses? Some of those that I interviewed—such as Nichani, health data sales experts, and those who work for data aggregators or compilers—took pity on this poor detective, and tried to guess where I might look. Most were intrigued that I was interested in learning about the work that they do, and were willing to share. When I told them that I was looking for my marketing baby, they were genuinely shocked and appalled to hear about my haunting and tried to figure out how it could have happened. My mystery became theirs as well.

Maybe you filled out a survey online? Did you tell anyone on Facebook that you were pregnant? Did someone email congratulations to you? Maybe someone in the doctor's office leaked out the information? Some told me that I would never find what I was looking for because the system has firewalls in place and my data could never come back to haunt me. Others explained that personal identifying information, especially concerning someone's health or financial information, is siloed and quarantined, and thus could not be used to target a specific consumer. That's not how the system works, they said. How it is supposed to work, they relayed, is that the data of millions of consumers is aggregated and segmented into large datasets. There is supposedly no algorithmic way to drill down to an identifiable individual. Still others told me that a payment made by credit card at my doctor's office, for instance, cannot be "seen" by my issuing bank, and anyway, all of the data is de-identified and anonymized; there is no possibility that any could leak out or be reconnected to me. The data, they said, is secure. Yet, there I stood before these data-marketing professionals as living proof that the system is *built to identify me*, to rematerialize my data into a living, breathing commodity.

This is why I found it so surprising that when I relayed my personal story of being haunted by my own data, these insiders expressed shock and were sincerely appalled that I was marketed to in such a way. I imagined that this was the first time they were confronted with a living, breathing human being that was directly affected by their target marketing efforts. I was not an anonymous or abstract dataset of a million customers. I was a single individual that was re-identified and marketed to based on an inferred health status: a pregnancy with a due date dreamed up algorithmically.

Although I didn't find a way to reassemble the body of my marketing baby (yes, I knew it was a futile pursuit. After all, this was a noir detective story.), I came a little closer to the origins of its conception, and I found comrades in my quest. I also found a much more interesting story. The story of my marketing baby became a story about a machine-controlled network of data and disclosure where the human agents who are tasked with its stewardship don't understand all of the ways that data is coming together and being used. They know how it is *supposed* to work, yet not how it really does work. This means that the story they tell themselves—the social imaginary that they use to collectively construct this network of lively data—enables them to trust that the system works, that something like what happened to me is not *supposed* to happen (Taylor 2003). This big black box of data, in which really smart people try to innovate on and gain insights from that data, somehow has become an autonomous "data machine" with its own agency—a golem stomping around the countryside, wreaking havoc. Through standing face-to-face with these industry insiders and sharing my story of trauma wrought by *dumb* data, I was able to humanize data commodities. In my sharing, I found empathy, not a defense of the data marketing industry as I had expected that I would find. In fact, I realized that I have more comrades than I had imagined, and even managed to recruit a few more detectives onto the case. Ultimately, however, I found that we are all algorithmic subjects. As Natasha Dow Schüll demonstrates in her book *Addiction by Design*, a 20-year ethnographic study of the gaming industry, surveillance and data collection technologies work in confluence with architecture, algorithms, and pharmacology to produce a "whirring assemblage" that suspends players in the "machine zone," a zone that ensnares players with psychological rewards to encourage more game playing by providing always-unfulfilled hope and encouraging risk taking (Schüll 2012). Similarly, big data becomes a black box that ensnares all of us—database marketers and consumers alike—into a "whirring assemblage" of algorithms, data, and marketing. Big data is a black box for the insiders that construct the box as much as it is for the subjects of the black box.

Notes

1. I am using the actual name of the Request Initiative lawyer, with his kind permission. Before going to the &Then DMA convention, I had worked with the Request Initiative, a UK-based data rights organization, to track down my marketing baby. I recruited Request Initiative onto the case for three reasons: The organization's modus operandi is to make data subject requests as a way of pressuring government and corporations to be transparent about the data they hold on people; Experian is, ostensibly, an European Union (EU) company headquartered in Dublin, and therefore beholden to EU and UK data subject laws; and finally, due to the more stringent EU data laws, Request Initiative could submit a data subject access request directly to a company, with the backing of UK and EU data rights legislation. While the organization, and especially Samir, worked hard to help me obtain my data, in the end, we could not get anything out of Experian other than a credit report and an "opt-out" form for credit card offers.
2. When I approached the representatives working at the Experian exhibition booth, they refused to speak to me, once I explained to them that I was a sociologist conducting fieldwork on how data brokers use health data. While I found this frustrating and disappointing, it was also hardly surprising to me that this would happen. In fact, this was the only time during all of my fieldwork for this project where I was refused an interview with industry professionals. So, the explosive showdown that I fantasized about turned out to be a dud—it fizzled.
3. During interviews with data brokers at the trade show, most used golf as an example of an inferred sports interest. Golf, of course, is a sport that has certain race, gender, and class implications that indicated what kind of customer brokers have in mind when targeting them.

4. I found these mantras on the banners and trade show booths for Epsilon Data Management LLC, Teradata Corp., and Infogroup. They also appear on these companies' websites and other promotional materials. The marketing refrains show how the industry understands how data can serve clients who are trying to procure or retain customers, and ultimately increase revenue.
5. First Data and Chase Paymentech are both payment processing and merchant services companies.

References

BenMark, Gadi, and Masri Maher. 2015. "Cracking the Digital-Shopper Genome." *McKinsey.com*, August. Accessed January 26, 2016. http://www.mckinsey.com/insights/marketing_sales/cracking_the_digital-shopper_genome.

Direct Marketing Association. 2015. *&Then Event Guide*. New York: Direct Marketing Association.

Eichelberger, Erika. 2014. "10 Things Elizabeth Warren's Consumer Protection Agency Has Done for You." *Mother Jones*, March 14. Accessed January 26, 2016. http://www.motherjones.com/politics/2014/02/elizabeth-warren-consumer-financial-protection-bureau.

Experian Marketing Services. 2009. "Mosaic® USA: Consumer Lifestyle Segmentation for the United States." Experian Marketing Services. https://www.experian.com/assets/marketing-services/product-sheets/mosaic-usa.pdf.

———. 2015. *Mapping Your Customer's DNA: A CMO Imperative*. New York: Experian Marketing Services. http://www.experian.com/marketing-services/single-customer-view-ebook.html.

———. 2016. *Demonstrate the Importance of a Single Customer View*. New York: Experian Marketing Suite. http://www.experian.com/marketing-services/single-customer-view-worksheet.html.

Fair Isaac Corporation. 2012. "From Big Data to Big Marketing: Seven Essentials." FICO® INSIGHTS White Paper 63. San Jose, CA: Fair Isaac.

Hayles, N. Katherine. 1999. *How We Became Posthuman: Virtual Bodies in Cybernetics, Literature, and Informatics*. Chicago: University of Chicago Press.

Jennings, Andrew. 2015. "A Day in the Analytic Life of a Credit Card." FICO® White Paper. San Jose, CA: IMPACT the OR Society.

Merchant, Carolyn. 2008. "Secrets of Nature: The Bacon Debates Revisited." *Journal of the History of Ideas* 69 (1): 147–62.

Robert, Don. 2013. "Investor Seminar—January 2013." Investor Seminar report. London: Experian plc.

Schüll, Natasha Dow. 2012. *Addiction by Design: Machine Gambling in Las Vegas*. Princeton, NJ: Princeton University Press.

Solove, Daniel J. 2006a. *The Digital Person: Technology and Privacy in the Information Age*. New York: New York University Press.

———. 2006b. "A Taxonomy of Privacy." *University of Pennsylvania Law Review* 154 (3): 477–564.

Steel, Emily. 2011. "Using Credit Cards to Target Web Ads." *Wall Street Journal*, October 25. Accessed January 26, 2016. http://www.wsj.com/articles/SB10001424052970204002304576627030651339352.

Taylor, Charles. 2003. *Modern Social Imaginaries*. Durham, NC and London: Duke University Press.

Thacker, Eugene. 2003a. "Data Made Flesh: Biotechnology and the Discourse of the Posthuman." *Cultural Critique* 53: 72–97.

———. 2003b. "What Is Biomedia?" *Configurations* 11 (1): 47–79.

CHAPTER 8

Life After Death

Like all good noirs, this hard-boiled tale, this dark quest for knowledge, was doomed from the start. My object of pursuit, my marketing baby, was nothing more than an apparition, a phantom, though one that pointed to a much bigger but infinitely unknowable conspiracy. Like most noirs, this one has an ambiguous and inconclusive ending.

The closing scene in my search found this detective sitting at a dimly lit desk in a darkened office, my head—crowned with a fresh crop of gray hairs, earned through the dogged pursuit of a tenacious specter—hovered over the final piece of evidence: a four-page letter from Experian. Rubbing my weary eyes, I read the company's boiler-plate prose:

> Thank you for your recent inquiry to Experian. Your privacy is very important to us and we want to provide you with a clear understanding of the type of information that may be contained in our marketing database. The information is used by companies and non-profit organizations to provide you with offers that may be relevant and of interest to you.
>
> This marketing data summary describes the type of information related to your household that has been collected by Experian and is maintained in Experian's marketing database. Experian obtains information from a number of public and proprietary sources, as described below, and uses quality control procedures to help identify inaccurate or out-of-date information. ... You can be confident that the data compilation process at Experian not only complies with state and federal laws, but also is developed with careful consideration of both past and anticipated privacy legislation and public opinion. ... As a leader in the direct-marketing industry, Experian strives to

M.F.E. Ebeling, *Healthcare and Big Data*,
DOI 10.1057/978-1-137-50221-6_8

> achieve a balance between consumer privacy expectations and our clients' business needs to ensure that both benefit. (Experian Marketing Services 2015, p. 1)

The letter did not describe further the public and proprietary data sources as promised, but the footer of each page was emblazoned with the phrase: "Experian confidential and proprietary." I read the following three pages with some incredulity, tinged with resignation. Known and Inferred Age: 40–49; Inferred Gender: Female; Estimated Education: Graduate Degree; Known and Inferred Presence of Children: Yes.

I put the letter down. No birth date for my marketing baby? No inferred gender? No known or inferred health status or "interests"? (Although, how can a data revenant have a health status…a dead thing reanimated by segmentation studies and algorithms?)

That was it. Like the shadow that vaporizes into a steamy dark alley, my marketing baby disappeared into the darkness of databases.

The Uncanny Life of Data

What kind of life does data take on without us? My investigation for this book led me to follow the data trails that possibly could lead back to my marketing baby. For four years, I have pursued the data that I produced in the fertility clinic, data that was captured by the network of disclosure through my electronic health record and through the prescription information written for me by Dr. Gaonkar. After it was stripped of my identifying information, my data was most certainly sold to third parties. My procedural data was sent to my health insurer for reimbursement, as was all of the transactional data that was produced from the $25,000 that I charged to my credit card to pay for the in vitro fertilization (IVF) expenses not covered by my insurance. Additionally, I participated in a clinical trial and the data that my body produced while under study was certainly captured digitally and disclosed to the sponsor of the clinical study and used to promote the success of the study drug. Presumably, all of this data, some of it de-identified, some of it not, ended up in Experian's data warehouses where it was recombined with "public and proprietary" data sources—my house's deed and mortgage, my online browser behaviors, my retail pharmacy purchases of ovulation detection and pregnancy tests. With this, data brokers developed a data marketing image of me as an individual, pregnant consumer and sold that data marketing "me" onwards as a data commodity.

Having little success meeting my marketing baby face-to-face, despite enlisting the help of Request Initiative data and human rights lawyer Samir Dathi, asking data brokers at the &Then data marketing trade show in Boston, and repeatedly phoning, emailing, and sending requests directly to Experian, I held on to one last hope: submitting a complaint with the Consumer Financial Protection Bureau (CFPB). Perhaps, by filing a complaint against Experian Marketing Services with the heft of a governmental organization behind me, this grizzled gumshoe might finally come face-to-face with my data revenant, my marketing baby.

I tracked down the online complaint form, where I can choose to lodge a grievance with a credit bureau. With some trepidation (I have grown quite "data paranoid" during this investigation), I completed it. I wrote that my core complaint was that I received unsolicited marketing based on my health data and tracked down the origins of the direct marketing to Experian. The last part of the form asked about my desired outcome. Here is what I wrote:

> **Question 3: Desired Resolution**
>
> I want detailed, accurate information on all of my personal data held, all of the data sources that were used, and all of the marketing segments and products that my data was funneled into by Experian Marketing Services.
>
> For example, Experian Marketing Services has a segmentation platform called MOSAIC, and they claim to hold data on 98 percent of American households within this product and have categorized all of us based on our gender, race, income, the value of property we may own, where we live, what diseases we may have, and so on. They sell these segmentation studies through their Marketing Services. I would like to know, through this product, how my personal data is segmented. I want to SEE how I am characterized, what kind of data image Experian sells about my life, especially about my health. So a fair resolution for me would be for me to take POSSESSION of all of my own data, all of the details of my life that Experian claims to 'own' and which, based on this ownership claim, 'sells' to an unknown number of people, through their marketing services products.
>
> Furthermore, I want to know about every single data source that Experian Marketing Services uses to collect data on me. According to my discussions with ALC, for example, Experian claims to use forty data sources to construct the '*Newborn Network*' list, and Experian claims that those sources are 'proprietary information.' I would like the name of each data source and to know exactly which of my data came from which source. And beyond the particular Newborn Network product, I would like to know exactly all of the data sources and what kinds of data are used for other marketing

> services within Experian. Finally, I want to know exactly how much data as well as what kinds of data are shared between the credit bureau services and the marketing services portions of the Experian business. Are data that is collected from mortgage applications or credit card transactions by the credit bureau shared or used by the data marketing services or by MOSAIC? I want to see every bit of data that has been shared and made into a product.
>
> I would also like to know how much money Experian has made off of my data, how much financial value has my trauma and suffering produced for Experian Marketing Services? I want a dollar figure on my pain. That, for me, would be a fair resolution..

I clicked the "Submit" button. Immediately, I felt lighter, less burdened. They couldn't ignore me now, I thought. I had finally had my say on precisely what I wanted from Experian: for the data broker to give me back what they took from me and to recognize that their acquisition of my data was my dispossession, that they profit on the suffering of millions of faceless, but not nameless, consumers.

I waited.

Six weeks later, I received another unsolicited credit report and an opt-out form for credit card offers.

From the Black Box to the Databased Society

What are the logics of a society that is rendered at the same time visible and invisible through the database? One in which life is disassembled into component and corresponding bits, to produce more value than the whole. In such a society, all qualities of human life, of existence, are quantified, cut up, digitized, and reassembled to take on new lives and new meanings that are barely recognizable from the original sources.

Throughout this detective's tale, like in many noir narratives, the search for the truth led a detective down unforeseen paths and entrapped her in some unexpected warrens. Although it may not have produced the truth about my marketing baby per se, my investigation nonetheless produced several truths about our uncanny data lives in the databased society. As patients, we do not give our informed consent to the collection, use, and disclosure of our health data. In the databased society, both patients and health practitioners alike are produced as biocapital data subjects by the network of disclosure. We are all produced by and simultaneously produce the network. While we may be the producers of valuable health data, we do not own that data. Instead, data innovators and holders claim ownership.

It is no accident that on each page of the Consumer Marketing Report sent to me by Experian Marketing Services, the data broker branded itself the proprietor of my data. It is not mine; it is theirs. This, of course, underlines the asymmetrical power relations of data. We can resist and we do in a variety of ways, perhaps most obviously when patients submit a data breach complaint to the Department of Health and Human Services (HHS)'s Office of Civil Rights—but to do so, patients need to know that their data has been breached in the first place. In many regards, doctors and nurses are very cognizant of protecting and respecting the privacy rights of their patients; they see it as part of the overall quality of care that they provide. Yet, they similarly are subjects of the network of disclosure, of the databased society, as much as patients are. Healthcare providers have very limited control over what happens to patient data beyond their individual, day-to-day, vigilant privacy practices. Although we have some control over our data, most of that power is asymmetrically skewed toward those who claim ownership of data, and that isn't us. Data breach complaints address one node in a complex network, but at any point our data can be breached—legally. As I have shown in this book, we need to concern ourselves with the normative precedents laid down by the data brokerage industry, the "business-as-usual" disclosures and commodification of health data. If a data privacy and legal scholar like Helen Nissenbaum (2010), who has dedicated her career to studying how data surveillance operates, says that she doesn't know how all of our data is collected and used, if she can't keep up with the algorithms that control our lives, what hope do we—who have less time, money, social capital, and resources—have of turning this boat around and gaining some control?

In her book *Dark Matters* (Browne 2015), mentioned in Chapter 1, Simone Browne proposes a political project in regard to biometric data, the data that are connected to our bodies but used by the security and surveillance state to profile us, to assess the level of danger and risk associated with our bodies, with our features, with what she calls, borrowing from Frantz Fanon, our "epidermalization" threat level. She shows how the social meanings of race are traced, or as Browne persuasively demonstrates, are *branded*, onto our skin by biometric technologies. Browne argues that we must develop a "critical biometric consciousness," similar to what Eugene Thacker proposes with genomic data, one in which the public are engaged in informed debates over the use of their biologically derived data (Thacker 2003a, b). She also calls for the creation of state and private accountability systems in which access to and ownership of data produced by people's bodies is a right of the data producers—us—and not of the data innovators (Browne 2015, p. 116). There are patient and data rights activists that are working on this very proposal. Take, for example, Hugo Campos, who has fought for his rights over the data produced by his heart through his pacemaker implanted in his body, or the patients who upload their medical and health data to Patientslikeme.com, where instead of losing control over the use and disclosure of their data in the network of disclosure, these patients crowd source, open source, and redefine, on their own terms, the value of their data.

In his book *The Black Box Society: The Secret Algorithms That Control Money and Information* (2015), Frank Pasquale argues that the network of disclosure, where our data is scraped by data brokers to steal this value, characterizes a black box society, where capitalism uses "automated processes to assess risk and allocate opportunity" through a proprietary and algorithmic logic of secrecy, dispossession, and ownership (Pasquale 2015, p. 216). He notes that this secrecy has produced system-wide trauma and harm:

> [B]ad information is as likely to endure as good, and to result in unfair and even disastrous [outcomes]. This is why the wholesale use of black box modeling, however profitable it is for the insiders who manage it, is dangerous to society as a whole. It's bad enough when innocent individuals are hurt, branded as security threats or goldbrickers or credit risks or by inaccuracies that they can't contest and not even know about. …. Moreover, when the errors are systematic enough, algorithmic control fails on its own terms. Educated citizenship today requires more than an understanding of government … it also demands an understanding of the companies that influence our government and culture … [corporations that] increasingly determine the value and visibility of labor, companies and investments. (2015, pp. 216–217)

Pasquale contends that if we do not, as a society, move away from what he calls the black box society to the intelligible society, power will always skew toward those who own the algorithms, those who own the databases, those who own our data. As with Schüll's "whirring assemblage" built by the gaming industry that ensnares gamblers in a pharmacotechnological trap, similarly, the databased society ensnares people through a confluence of database architectures, incentives, rewards, and bargains that are always skewed against us; they are never deals that benefit us (Schüll 2012).

What kind of society are we making for ourselves when every aspect of our lives is spliced up into data bits, drained of vitality, rendered, boiled down, and reassembled into commodities that produce value for those who hold the keys to the black box in the first place? This book has taken up Pasquale's demand to open the black box of the databased society, to expose the structures of power undergirding the data industry. Yet, my investigation also shows that it is not enough to simply expose the algorithms to make it intelligible. We also need to question what kind of databased society are we constructing in the first place. We need to not only question, but to refuse our consent every time we are asked to hand over our data to feed into the machine.

The Noir Ending

Like all good noirs, though, I bring the conclusion of this detective story to an indeterminate and inconclusive end. What I can say, here, at the end, is that while I didn't find my marketing baby—in many ways I always knew that it was a futile search—I found a much more interesting story. In his lyrical film *Nostalgia for the Light*, filmmaker Patricio Guzmán presents a mediation on state violence, time, and loss, told through interviews with astronomers, archeologists, and prisoners who all share in the trauma and silence of Chile's recent past. During the film, Guzmán focuses his lens on a group of women who have, for close to thirty years, painstakingly searched, by hand, the Atacama desert for the bones of their loved ones who "disappeared" there during the Pinochet regime. Through the decades, these women have grown old; they are grayer and a bit more frail. While their bodies are bent, they are sloped downwards not with age, but with their constant searching of the desert's parched ground. Guzmán's interviews Vicky Saavedra about her hunt for the bones of her brother José struck a deep vein of recognition in me, and pulled at my heart. Saavedra describes the relentless aching and agony that drives her search, knowing that her brother's body is dispersed among the ancient rocks. Saavedra explains that when she finally found her brother's foot during the excavation of a mass grave—she knew it was his foot from the color of the sock and shoe—she held that one piece of him and cried. Eventually, she placed his foot on her mantelpiece and every evening she takes it down and gently cradles it, not as an object of death but as an uncanny thing enlivened through her tears and love with José's life force. Despite this macabre reunion—one that brings Saavedra no resolution and no peace—after 28 years of combing the sand for bone fragments, Saavedra tells the filmmaker that she will not stop searching the desert floor until she has assembled the entirety of her brother's body.

While my losses or my anticipated reunion with my marketing baby in no way can compare to Saavedra's story of loss through genocidal violence, there is something in what she describes that resonates with me. I, too, have an abiding need to reassemble the pieces into a whole, into a body, to reanimate the life that was connected to my own body. My marketing baby and I are part of a kinship network that stretches into the past and future. Yet, my marketing baby was torn from me to become a corpse. I understand the desire for a reunion with the uncanny thing made alive again.

References

Browne, Simone. 2015. *Dark Matters: On the Surveillance of Blackness.* Durham, NC: Duke University Press.

Experian Marketing Services. 2015. "Consumer Marketing Report." EBELING, MARY F. New York: Experian Marketing Services.

Nissenbaum, Helen. 2010. Privacy in Context: Technology, Policy, and the Integrity of Social Life. Palo Alto, CA: Stanford University Press.

Pasquale, Frank. 2015. *The Black Box Society: The Secret Algorithms That Control Money and Information.* Cambridge, MA: Harvard University Press.

Schüll, Natasha Dow. 2012. *Addiction by Design: Machine Gambling in Las Vegas.* Princeton, NJ: Princeton University Press.

Thacker, Eugene. 2003a. "Data Made Flesh: Biotechnology and the Discourse of the Posthuman." *Cultural Critique* 53: 72–97.

———. 2003b. "What Is Biomedia?" *Configurations* 11 (1): 47–79.

Index

Note: Bold page numbers refer to figures, page numbers followed by "n" refers to notes.

M.F.E. Ebeling, *Healthcare and Big Data*,
DOI 10.1057/978-1-137-50221-6